ATKINS DIET FOR BEGINNERS

Atkins Diet Cookbook, Atkins Low Carb Diet, Rapid Weight Loss

(Easy to Follow Atkins Diet Recipes)

Floyd Roberts

Published by Alex Howard

© Floyd Roberts

All Rights Reserved

Atkins Diet for Beginners: Atkins Diet Cookbook, Atkins Low Carb Diet, Rapid Weight Loss (Easy to Follow Atkins Diet Recipes)

ISBN 978-1-990169-63-2

All rights reserved. No part of this guide may be reproduced in any form without permission in writing from the publisher except in the case of brief quotations embodied in critical articles or reviews.

Legal & Disclaimer

The information contained in this book is not designed to replace or take the place of any form of medicine or professional medical advice. The information in this book has been provided for educational and entertainment purposes only.

The information contained in this book has been compiled from sources deemed reliable, and it is accurate to the best of the Author's knowledge; however, the Author cannot guarantee its accuracy and validity and cannot be held liable for any errors or omissions. Changes are periodically made to this book. You must consult your doctor or get professional medical advice before using any of the suggested remedies, techniques, or information in this book.

Table of contents

PART 1 1

INTRODUCTION 2

LIGHT N' LEAN BURGER W/ COLESLAW 8

EASY GAZPACHO "SMOOTHIE" 10

"TURKEY-TOUILLE" 11

LOW CARB BEEF STROGANOFF 13

GLUTEN FREE WAFFLES 15

LOW CARB MEXICAN CHILI 16

ZUCCHINI FLAX N' PROTEIN BREAD 18

ALMOND-RASPBERRY CUPCAKES 20

BBQ CHICKEN PIZZA W/SALAD 22

MEXICAN STUFFED PEPPERS 24

SALMON-ASPARAGUS CREPES 26

PANCETTA N' CABBAGE 28

LOW CAL INDIAN TIKKA CHICKEN 30

STUFFED TURKEY BREAST WITH ARUGULA SALAD 31

ZUCCHINI PANCAKES WITH FETA, WALNUTS AND OREGANO 33

TACO SALAD 35

SHRIMP GUMBO 37

ROAST BEEF AND MIXED GREENS WITH PICKLED OKRA AND RADISHES 39

PORK TENDERLOIN WITH TOMATOES AND GREEN OLIVES 40

PUMPKIN-SPICE BROWNIES 42

SPICY TURNIP FRIES 44

KALE CHIPS 45

HAM N' CHEESE FRITTATA 47

Roast Chicken And Vegetable Stew 50
Coconut-Almond Cookies 52
Camembert Cheese 54

PART 2 56

INTRODUCTION 57

CHAPTER 1: EVERY DIET STARTS WITH YOU! 59

CHAPTER 2: WHY THE ATKINS DIET? 64

CHAPTER 3: HOW THE ATKINS DIET WORKS 69

One Week Menu For Atkins 76
Chapter 4: Tips And Tricks To Be Successful 80
While On The Atkins Diet 80

CHAPTER 5: BREAKFAST RECIPES 88

One Minute Coconut And Almond Muffins 88
Pineapple-Almond Smoothie 89
Almond And Blueberry Pancakes 90
Jack Cheese, Avocado And Bacon Omelets With Freshly Made Salsa 92

CHAPTER 6: LUNCH RECIPES 94

Macho Chili 94

CHAPTER 7: DINNER RECIPES 96

Apricot Glazed Brisket 96
Bacon Wrapped Filet With Blue Cheese Butter Sauce 98
Chapter 8: Dessert Recipes 100
Raspberry-Almond Cupcakes 100
Atkins Brownies 102
Chocolate Ginger Cake 103

CHAPTER 9: ENTREE RECIPES 106

Almond-Raspberry Cupcakes 106

Apricot-Glazed Brisket 108

Artichokes With Lemon-Butter 109

Arugula, Pear And Hazelnut Salad 111

Asian Beef Salad With Edamame 112

Asian Beef Salad With Sesame Seeds 114

Asian Lobster Salad 115

Asian Marinade 116

Asian Steak Salad 117

Asian Tuna Kebabs 119

Asian Vegetable Bowl 120

Asian Veggie And Pork Bowl 121

Asian-Style Coleslaw 123

Asparagus And Leek Soup 124

Asparagus In Vinaigrette With Walnuts 125

Asparagus Tarragon Cream Soup 126

Asparagus Wrapped In Chili Spiced Bacon 127

Asparagus, Mushrooms And Peas 128

Atkins Chocolate Slushies 130

Atkins Cinnamon Pie Crust 131

Atkins Coconut Layer Cake 132

Atkins Cuisine Brownies 133

Atkins Cuisine Cookies 134

Atkins Cuisine Pizza With Sausage, Bell Peppers And Onions 136

Atkins Cuisine Pizza-Barbecue Chicken Supreme 138

Atkins Yorkshire Pudding 139

Avocado Gazpacho Smoothie 140

Avocado Zucchini Soup	141
Baby Greens With Grapefruit And Red Onion	142
Baby Spinach, Pickled Beets And Tomato Salad	144
Bacon And Goat Cheese Salad	145
Bacon Wrapped Filet With Blue Cheese Butter Sauce	146
Bacon-Egg Salad Flatout Wrap	148
Bahian Halibut	149
Baked Artichoke-Parsley Cheese Squares	150
Baked Catfish With Broccoli And Herb-Butter Blend	151
Baked Chicken With Artichokes	152
Baked Fennel Au Gratin	154
Baked Goat Cheese And Ricotta Custards	155
Baked Meatballs	156
Baked Quesadillas	157
Baked Red Bell Peppers Filled With Cherry Tomatoes And Feta	159
Baked Salmon With Bok Choy And Mixed Greens	160
Baked Salmon With Bok Choy And Red Bell Pepper Purée	161
Baked Tamari-Lemon Pork Chops	163
Baked Tofu With Asian Marinade	164
Baked Tofu With Cajun Rub	164
Baked Tofu With Chipotle Marinade	165
Baked Tofu With Latin Marinade	166
Baked Tofu With Mediterranean Marinade	167
Baked Tofu With Moroccan Rub	168
Baked Tofu With Red Bell Pepper, Broccoli And Peanut Sauce	169
Balsamic Pork Loin And Cauliflower	170
Barbecue Rub	171
Barbecue Sauce	172
Barbecued Glazed Ham	174

Basic Custard Ice Cream	175
Basic Egg Salad	176
Basic Steamed Lobster With Drawn Butter	177
Basic Tomato Sauce	178
Basil Pesto	179
Bearnaise Sauce	180
Béchamel Sauce	181
Beef And Vegetable Stew	182
Beef Bolognaise With Parmesan	184
Beef Burger With Feta And Tomato	185
Beef Carpaccio With Arugula And Caper Vinaigrette	186
Beef Fajitas With Peppers	187
Beef Fillet With Bacon And Gorgonzola Butter	Error! Bookmark not defined.
Beef Fondue	Error! Bookmark not defined.
Beef Sautéed With Green Bell Pepper And Onions Topped With Cheese	Error! Bookmark not defined.
Beef Sauteed With Vegetables Over Romaine	Error! Bookmark not defined.
Beef Stroganoff	Error! Bookmark not defined.
Beef Tenderloin	Error! Bookmark not defined.
Beef, Scallions And Red Bell Pepper Sauté	Error! Bookmark not defined.
Bittersweet Chocolate Brownie Drops	Error! Bookmark not defined.
Blackberry Clafouti	Error! Bookmark not defined.
Blackberry Spinach Salad With Goat Cheese Medallions	Error! Bookmark not defined.
Blackened Salmon With Cucumber Relish And Cauliflower	Error! Bookmark not defined.
Blender Mayonnaise	Error! Bookmark not defined.
Blue Cheese And Bacon Soup	Error! Bookmark not defined.
Blue Cheese Dressing	Error! Bookmark not defined.

BLUEBERRY-CUCUMBER CHILLER .... ERROR! BOOKMARK NOT DEFINED.
BLUEBERRY-TURKEY BURGERS .... ERROR! BOOKMARK NOT DEFINED.
BOK CHOY AND GREEN ONIONS .... ERROR! BOOKMARK NOT DEFINED.
BONES-TO-BE CHICKEN WINGETTES .... ERROR! BOOKMARK NOT DEFINED.
BOUILLABAISSE .... ERROR! BOOKMARK NOT DEFINED.
BRAISED LEEKS AND FENNEL .... ERROR! BOOKMARK NOT DEFINED.
BRATWURST WITH ONIONS AND SAUERKRAUT .... ERROR! BOOKMARK NOT DEFINED.
BRATWURST WITH SAUERKRAUT .... ERROR! BOOKMARK NOT DEFINED.

CONCLUSION **189**

Part 1

Introduction

The Atkins diet is a popular low-carbohydrate system of eating that was created by cardiologist Robert C. Atkins in 1972. It has been updated and revised over the past several decades, but the main ideals have remained the same. The Atkins diet declares that the reason for our weight gain, the root cause of the obesity epidemic is not overconsumption of fats and proteins, but rather carbohydrates and refined grains. The Atkins diet has helped millions of people lose unwanted pounds, and it has spurred an influx of other low-carb diets such as the South Beach diet, Paleo diet, and the Sonoma diet. But how exactly does eating less carbs and more fatty foods, the cornerstone idea of the Atkins diet, help you to lose weight?

Simply put, by eliminating carbs from the diet, completely in the first weight loss stages of the diet but still heavily restricted in later maintenance phases of the diet, it forces the body's metabolic systems to switch from metabolizing glucose for energy to using stored fats for energy, a process known as ketosis. This helps us to lose weight quickly and easily as the body is consuming its own stored fat reserves for energy, depleting and eliminating the excess fatty tissue.

Eating a low carb diet also helps you to lose weight because it suppresses the appetite. This may be due to the fact that it takes the body longer to digest fats, proteins, and fiber-rich foods, all of which are featured in Atkins. This means that it takes longer for you to feel hungry. Also, the fulfilling nature of the fat-rich foods, proteins, and fibers makes you feel more satisfied overall.

Think about it, if you're allowed to eat a nice sized, fatty steak, you're going to feel more satisfied than if you pick at a tiny portion of rice. Many people find success with the Atkins diet because they are allowed to eat more filling, fatty foods that don't feel like diet foods at all.

Another popular plus for the Atkins plan is the fact that you don't have to count calories. The only metric that you must track is overall net carb consumption. To do this, you simply take the total carb content of an item and subtract the fiber content. For example, a half cup of broccoli has 2.3 grams of total carbs but 1.3 grams of fiber, making net carb content only 1 gram. Different phases of the diet allow different net carb consumption levels, but they typically range from 20 net carbs to 50 or more, depending on your body weight.

Preferred foods on the Atkins diet include all sources of meat, eggs, cheese, vegetables, and oils. Whole, unprocessed versions of each food source are preferred, at least one source of protein should accompany every meal. Vegetables should be those with lower glycemic indexes, or lower net carb scores, and the most popular vegetables for those following the Atkins diet are asparagus, broccoli, celery, cucumbers, green beans, and bell peppers. After the initial weight-loss phase of the diet, fruits, starchy veggies, and some natural whole grains can also be included.

The Atkins diet succeeds for many people because it includes many delicious, fulfilling foods that make the plan seem less like a diet and more like a lifestyle change. The ability to eat fatty foods and a variety of proteins makes the diet extremely appealing to many new dieters, and not having to count every single calorie can make the plan easier to follow. As you progress with the diet, adding back some carbs such as fruits and whole grains makes the plan feel balanced and manageable, and many, many people have found success through healthier lives with this unique plan.

History

The Atkins diet is the brainchild of Dr. Robert Atkins. Born in Columbus, Ohio in 1930, he received his medical degree from Cornell University and completed a cardiology residency at Columbia University. He then opened his own medical practice specializing in cardiology and complementary medicine in New York City in 1959, but his new, stressful, metropolitan lifestyle led to weight gain. After reading research completed by Dr. Alfred W. Pennington regarding the use of diets restricting sugars and starches, he lost a considerable amount of weight, and he began recommending this type of diet to many of his patients. In 1965 he appeared on **The Tonight Show** to discuss his low-carb eating plan, and his recommendations were published in **Vogue** magazine, leading many to call Dr. Atkin's early plan "The Vogue Diet." Realizing the popularity of his diet and the effective of the plan for many of his patients and followers, Atkins published his own book, **Dr. Atkins' Diet Revolution** in 1972. The book flew off the shelves and became an instant bestseller. This first book led to many other products produced under the Atkins brand, products such as low-glycemic snack bars, shakes, cookbooks, supplements, and other lifestyle items. In 1992, he revised his diet by publishing **Dr. Atkins' New Diet Revolution**. In this updated version there is more focus on eating nutritious foods and not just low-carb foods, although the basic principles of forcing the body into ketosis is the same. This revised edition sold over 15 million copies in the United States alone, and sparked a low-carb craze that included the publication and popularity of other, similar low-carb diet concepts. Dr. Atkins died in 2003, but his legacy lives on in the numerous products and books that bare his name and his specialized dieting plan that has helped so many lose weight.

Benefits

Cutting Carbs

The cornerstone of the Atkins diet is cutting out carbohydrates. Weight loss results as the body switches to burning its own fat reserves rather than calories from sugar, but cutting out those carbs actually has far reaching benefits beyond just dropping a few pounds of belly fat. By reducing carbohydrates, most people will see a marked reduction in triglycerides as fructose is the main driver of elevated levels of this dangerous substance in the body. High triglyceride levels are associated with strong heart disease factors, and by eliminating carbs, you can reduce your overall risk of heart disease, heart attack, and stroke caused by elevated triglyceride levels. Reducing carbs can also reduce the risk or severity of type II diabetes. Type II diabetes is caused by insulin resistance. The body fails to secrete enough insulin to fully absorb all the sugars in the blood, sugars that come directly from carbs in the diet, and this wreaks havoc on the body. Symptoms include dehydration, diabetic coma, and damage to the nerves, kidneys, heart, and eyes, leading to further medical complications. By not eating carbohydrates, you're reducing your body's need for insulin and lowering the risk of these symptoms occurring. Lowering carbohydrates can drastically reduce risk of heart disease and other serious ailments in addition to weight loss, and many of Dr. Atkins' patients were able to quit taking their diabetes and heart medications due to the health improvements they saw while on this plan.

Protein Power

While the Atkins diet is not a high-protein diet (simply a low-carb diet), protein is encouraged at every meal to maintain satiety and energy levels throughout the day. Protein is an important component to good health. It contains the building blocks required to construct and maintain bones, muscles, cartilage, skin, and blood as well as hormones, enzymes, and vitamins produced within the body. Without enough protein, these things cannot be properly produced or maintained and can lead to weakness, lethargy, and depression. Many meat-based sources of protein also contain iron, a very important nutrient that is required to carry oxygen to the blood. This allows the tissues of the entire body to remain properly nourished so that optimal functioning can occur. Iron deficiencies, or anemia, can result in fatigue, pale skin, abnormal heartbeat, shortness of breath, dizziness, and cognitive function issues. The Atkins plan ensures optimal levels of protein and iron, and this allows your body to work at its peak while feeling vital and energized.

Fats

Fats have become a bad word in the collective conscience of the average dieter, but in most cases, fats are not the main culprit. Fats are actually extremely important compounds that are essential to our bodies. The Atkins diet allows liberal use of fats, although more healthy unsaturated varieties are encouraged. Fats provide energy as they are the most efficient fuel sources available to our bodies, providing double the amount of available energy compared to carbs. Fats are also responsible for keeping our cells healthy as each cell contains a small amount of fat necessary for cushioning and protection, and they also help the body to absorb certain vitamins (A, D, E, and K) and use them more efficiently. Without fats in the diet, our bodies would not be able to function even on the cellular level. By eating dietary fats from natural, healthy sources, we provide our bodies with the important compounds it needs to continue these vital functions.

Cautions

Many people get overly excited when they hear there is no calorie counting with the Atkins diet and no restrictions on fats, meats, and cheeses. But overconsumption of any type of food can still lead to obesity and the many complications associated with being overweight. Exercise proper portion control with any diet, even the Atkins plan.

When the Atkins diet first hit the public scene in the 1960s and again in the 1990s with its republication and re-popularization, there were as many critics as supports. Many people have warned against a low-carb diet high in proteins and fats. Concerns arise from the consumption of animal products, meats, cheeses, milk, and yogurt, that are commonly consumed on the Atkins plan. These foods contain high levels of saturated fats and cholesterols, compounds that have been associated with high risk of heart attack and stroke, and also that can decrease overall bone mass while also increasing the risk of kidney stones and kidney failure. Many people are also concerned that leaving the body in a ketogenic state for long periods of time can be harmful, leading to kidney failure, diabetes, cancer, and even premature aging and death. While many of these claims are unsubstantiated, it is wise to take caution when beginning any new dietary regimen. Consult your doctor for the most up-to-date information on these concerns.

Light N' Lean Burger W/ Coleslaw

Time: 40 minutes

Serves: 1

Ingredients

¼ pound medium head of cabbage, halved and cored
1/8 cup fat-free mayonnaise
2 tablespoons fat-free sour cream
¼ tablespoon cider vinegar
1/8 tablespoon granular sugar substitute (sucralose)
1/8 teaspoon salt
1/8 teaspoon celery seed
6 ounces lean ground beef
1 ounce slice of fat free cheddar
½ Hass avocado, sliced
2 slices tomato

Directions

1. Cut cabbage into halves and thinly slice. Transfer to a large bowl.
2. In a small bowl, whisk together mayonnaise, sour cream, cider vinegar, sucralose, celery seed and salt. Mix the cabbage and dressing and refrigerate at least 30 minutes before serving for flavors to blend.
3. Preheat grill or broiler. Shape ground beef into a patty and season with salt and freshly ground black pepper. Cook about five minutes per side. Top with cheddar during last couple of minutes of cooking to melt the cheese. Add avocado and tomato to the burger and serve immediately with the coleslaw.

Nutritional Information

Serving Size: 446g, Calories: 607, Calories from Fat: 244, Total Fat: 27.1g, Saturated Fat: 6.8g, Cholesterol: 163, Sodium: 1037mg, Potassium: 1173mg, Total Carbs: 26.6g, Dietary Fiber: 7.2g, Sugars: 10.2g, Protein: 62.9g

Easy Gazpacho "Smoothie"

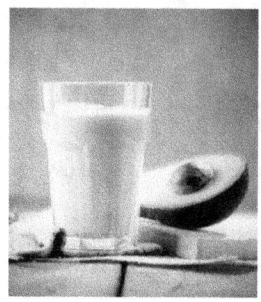

Time: 5 minutes

Serves: 1

Ingredients

1 Hass avocado, sliced
1 cup water
1 ounce reduced fat goat cheese
1 tablespoon fat free half and half
2 teaspoons freshly squeezed lime juice
2 teaspoons fresh chives, chopped
1/8 teaspoon salt

Directions

1. Purée avocado slices in a blender. Add water, goat cheese, half and half, lime juice, chives and salt and blend until

smooth. If needed, add additional water, one teaspoon at a time, to reach desired consistency.
2. Pour into a glass, and garnish with extra chives and an avocado slice, if desired. Serve chilled.

Nutritional Information

Serving Size: 572g, Calories: 519, Calories from Fat: 407, Total Fat: 45.3g, Saturated Fat: 12.4g, Cholesterol: 13, Sodium: 449mg, Potassium: 1093mg, Total Carbs: 26.5g, Dietary Fiber: 13.9g, Sugars: 3.8g, Protein: 9.5g

"Turkey-Touille"

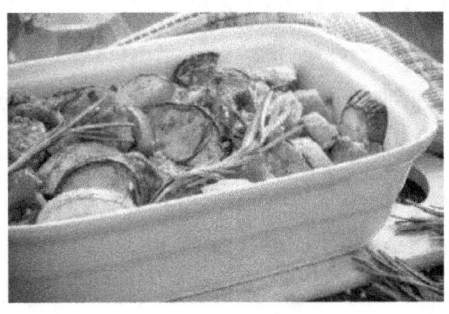

Time: 30 minutes

Serves: 4

Ingredients

4 tablespoons extra virgin olive oil, divided
24 ounces lean turkey breast cutlets
1 small eggplant, peeled and cut in 1-inch cubes
1 medium zucchini, trimmed and sliced
1 medium red bell pepper, seeded, cut in 1-inch pieces
1 cup trimmed, sliced button mushrooms
2 cloves garlic, minced
½ cup canned puréed tomatoes
1 teaspoon dried basil
½ teaspoon granular sugar substitute (sucralose)
1/8 teaspoon salt
1/8 teaspoon ground black pepper

Directions

1. Heat two tablespoons olive oil in a large skillet over medium heat. Sprinkle cutlets with salt and freshly ground black pepper. Sauté cutlets three minutes per side, just until lightly golden and cooked through. Transfer to a plate.
2. Heat remaining two tablespoons olive oil in skillet. Add eggplant, zucchini and red pepper. Sauté five minutes, stirring occasionally. Add mushrooms, garlic, tomato purée, basil and sugar substitute. Mix well; bring to a boil. Cover, reduce heat to low and simmer five minutes. Add salt and pepper to taste.
3. Return turkey and accumulated juices to skillet. Cook, uncovered two to three minutes, just until turkey is heated through.

4. Serve piping hot!

Nutritional Information
Serving Size: 428g, Calories: 357, Calories from Fat: 150, Total Fat: 16.7g, Saturated Fat: 2g, Cholesterol: 68mg, Sodium: 212mg, Potassium: 498mg, Total Carbs: 12.1g, Dietary Fiber: 6g, Sugars: 5.8g, Protein: 41.9g

Low Carb Beef Stroganoff

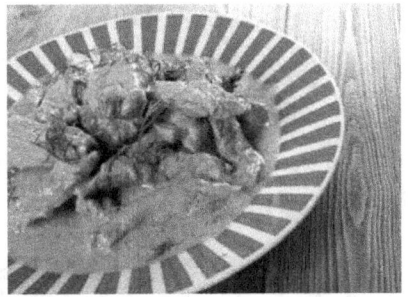

Time: 35 minutes

Serves: 4

Ingredients

1 ¼ pounds skirt steak, cut into 2- x 1-inch strips
1/8 teaspoon coarse sea salt
1/8 teaspoon pepper
2 tablespoons canola oil

1 tablespoon butter
½ cup finely chopped Spanish onion
3 ounces small white mushrooms
¼ cup dry red wine
1 cup beef broth (not low sodium)
¼ cup fat free sour cream
1 teaspoon Dijon mustard

Directions

1. Heat oven to warm setting. Season steak with salt and pepper.
2. Heat oil in a large non-stick skillet over medium-high heat. Brown meat in batches, about one minute per side. Transfer to a platter and place in oven.
3. Melt butter in skillet; add onion and sauté until soft and translucent. Add mushrooms. Cook 10 minutes, stirring occasionally, until mushroom liquid evaporates.
4. Add red wine; simmer 5 minutes. Stir in beef broth and simmer 10 more minutes, until mushrooms are coated with a thick sauce. Stir in sour cream and mustard. Add meat and accumulated juices.
5. Reduce heat to low and cook two to three minutes, until meat is heated through. Season to taste with salt and pepper.

Nutritional Information

Serving Size: 280g, Calories: 427, Calories from Fat: 221, Total Fat: 24.5g, Saturated Fat: 7.9g, Cholesterol: 93mg, Sodium: 410mg, Potassium: 509mg, Total Carbs: 5.3g, Dietary Fiber: 0.6g, Sugars: 1.9g, Protein: 40.5g

Gluten Free Waffles

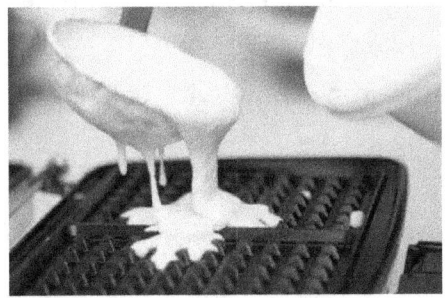

Time: 20 minutes

Serves: 5

Ingredients

1 cup gluten free All-Purpose Baking Mix
Olive oil cooking spray
1 packet granular sugar substitute
2 teaspoons baking powder
¼ teaspoon salt
1 cup fat free half and half
1 large egg

Directions

1. In a large bowl, mix together **baking mix**, baking powder, sugar substitute and salt.
2. In another large bowl, mix the half-and-half and beaten egg.
3. Add the ingredients from the two bowls together and whisk batter to remove any lumps. Do not overbeat.
4. Let the batter rest for at least five minutes to activate the baking powder.
5. Heat the waffle iron. Spray with cooking spray and pour in the batter using a ladle.
6. Close the top and cook waffles for about one to 1½ minutes or until golden brown.
7. Spray waffle iron with cooking spray in between each waffle.
8. Repeat until all the batter is used (makes five waffles).

Nutritional Information
Serving Size: 91g, Calories: 120, Calories from Fat: 9, Total Fat: 1g, Saturated Fat: 0g, Cholesterol: 37mg, Sodium: 756mg, Potassium: 215mg, Total Carbs: 23.4g, Dietary Fiber: 0.8g, Sugars: 5.7g, Protein: 2.1g

Low Carb Mexican Chili

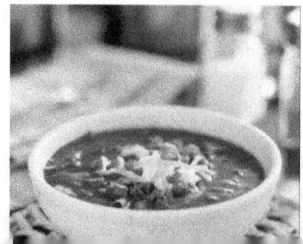

Time: 2 hours 45 minutes

Serves: 10

Ingredients

5 pounds boneless, lean beef chuck stew meat, cut in 1½ -inch cubes
2 teaspoons coarse sea salt
½ teaspoon freshly ground black pepper
3 tablespoons extra virgin olive oil
1 medium yellow onion, chopped
3 tablespoons ancho chili pepper powder or Mexican-style chili powder
1 (14½-ounce) can diced tomatoes with green chilies
¾ cup dry red wine
4 large roasted garlic cloves, minced
Shredded cheese (topping)
Sour cream (topping)
Green onion (topping)

Directions

1. Heat oven to 325°F.

2. Toss beef with salt and pepper. Heat 1½ teaspoon oil in a deep pan over high heat. Add one-third of the beef and brown on all sides, about five minutes.
3. Transfer to a bowl and repeat two more times with beef and oil.
4. Add the last 1½ teaspoons oil to the pan and cook onion until caramelized. Stir in chili powder, tomatoes, wine and garlic; bring to a simmer. Return beef and accumulated juices to the pan.
5. Cover and bake 2½ hours, stirring once halfway through cooking time, until beef is very tender.
6. Serve topped with shredded cheese, sour cream, and green onions.

Nutritional Information

Serving Size: 314g, Calories: 657, Calories from Fat: 457, Total Fat: 50.8g, Saturated Fat: 18.7g, Cholesterol: 161mg, Sodium: 763mg, Potassium: 764mg, Total Carbs: 4.6g, Dietary Fiber: 0.9g, Sugars: 2.3g, Protein: 38.9g

Zucchini Flax N' Protein Bread

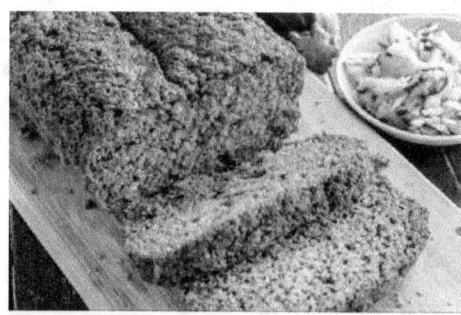

Time: 35 minutes

Serves: 6

Ingredients

2 large eggs
2 tablespoons extra virgin olive oil
1 teaspoon vanilla extract
1 cup shredded zucchini
1 cup golden flaxseed meal
2 tablespoons low-carb vanilla protein powder (1 ounce)
1/3 cup granular sugar substitute (sucralose)
¾ teaspoon baking powder
¼ teaspoon salt
1 ½ teaspoons ground cinnamon
1/8 teaspoon ground allspice
1/8 teaspoon nutmeg
Philadelphia cream cheese (topping)

Directions

1. Preheat an oven to 350°F. Grease six wells of a standard non-stick muffin tin.
2. Whisk eggs, oil and vanilla in a small bowl until frothy, about one minute. Add shredded zucchini.

3. Add flaxseed meal, protein powder, sugar substitute, baking powder, salt, and spices. Mix with a spoon to combine. Pour mix to fill ¾ of the muffin wells.
4. Bake for 25 minutes until slightly puffed, golden and cooked through. Enjoy with cream cheese.

Nutritional Information

Serving Size: 95g, Calories: 151, Calories from Fat: 111, Total Fat: 12.4g, Saturated Fat: 1.9g, Cholesterol: 62mg, Sodium: 123mg, Potassium: 139mg, Total Carbs: 6.8g, Dietary Fiber: 5.8g, Sugars: 0.6g, Protein: 6.3g

Almond-Raspberry Cupcakes

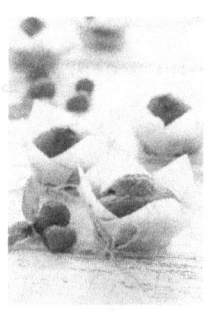

Time: 40 minutes

Serves: 10

Ingredients

2 large eggs (separated into whites and yolks)
¼ cup unsalted butter, softened
1/3 cup granular sugar substitute (sucralose)
2 tablespoons fat free half and half
2 tablespoons water
½ teaspoon freshly squeezed lemon juice
1 teaspoon vanilla extract
2 teaspoons almond extract
2 ½ cups almond flour
½ teaspoon baking powder
½ teaspoon salt
10 teaspoons sugar-free raspberry jam

Directions

1. Preheat oven to 350°F. Place 10 muffin or cupcake cups in a muffin pan and set aside. In a small bowl beat the egg yolks with ¼-cup sucralose, butter, half and half, water, lemon juice and almond extract until fully combined. Set aside.
2. In another bowl beat the egg whites until frothy, add the remaining two tablespoons of sucralose and continue to beat until stiff peaks form. Gently fold the egg whites into the egg-yolk mixture. Do not over-mix or the cupcakes will be too dense.
3. In a separate bowl, combine the almond meal, baking powder and salt. Gently fold into the egg mixture. Divide this batter equally between the muffin cups then drop one teaspoon of raspberry jam into the center of the batter.

4. Bake for 20 to 30 minutes until a toothpick inserted in the center comes out clean. Allow muffins to cool in the pan for five minutes and then take out and allow to cool on a cooling rack. Enjoy warm or at room temperature. Refrigerate remaining cupcakes in an airtight container for up to one week and serve at room temperature. These may also be frozen for up to one month.

Nutritional Information

Serving Size: 50g, Calories: 92, Calories from Fat: 72, Total Fat: 8g, Saturated Fat: 3.4g, Cholesterol: 49mg, Sodium: 170mg, Potassium: 76mg, Total Carbs: 3.1g, Dietary Fiber: 1.6g, Sugars: 0.7g, Protein: 2.3g

Bbq Chicken Pizza W/Salad

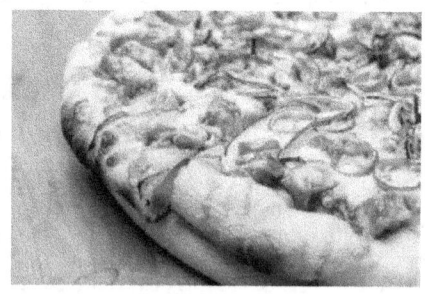

Time: 40 minutes

Serves: 8

Ingredients

2 cups gluten free All Purpose Low-Carb Baking Mix

1 **2/3** teaspoons baking powder

½ teaspoon salt

1 plus **1/16** packet granular sugar substitute (sucralose)

1 plus **1/16** (3 teaspoons) cup water

3 tablespoons plus 3 teaspoons extra virgin olive oil

4 ounces barbecue sauce

1 ½ cups shredded low fat mozzarella cheese

8 ounces cooked chicken breast, cut into ½-inch pieces

½ green bell pepper (thinly sliced)

1 red onion (thinly sliced)

12 cups shredded mixed greens

8 celery stalks (chopped)

40 cherry tomatoes

2 cups kidney beans

8 tablespoons light blue cheese Dressing

4 cups carrots, grated

Directions

1. Preheat oven to 425°F.
2. Blend flour, baking powder, salt and sugar in a large mixing bowl. Add water and oil with a spoon or spatula and combine into dough. With a spatula, take the dough out of the bowl and place on a clean surface lightly coated with non-stick vegetable oil spray.
3. Coat rolling pin with non-stick spray and roll the dough out to fit the pizza pan. It may be easier to use your hands.

4. Prebake crust for 10 minutes. Add barbecue sauce, mozzarella cheese, onions, bell pepper and chicken.
5. Continue baking at 425°F for 10 to 15 minutes.
6. Mix greens, celery, cherry tomatoes, kidney beans, carrots, and dressing. Serve with pizza on the side or on top!

Nutritional Information

Serving Size: 1179g, Calories: 815, Calories from Fat: 136, Total Fat: 15.1g, Saturated Fat: 2.5g, Cholesterol: 27mg, Sodium: 867mg, Potassium: 2902mg, Total Carbs: 135.3g, Dietary Fiber: 28.6g, Sugars: 33.1g, Protein: 37g

Mexican Stuffed Peppers

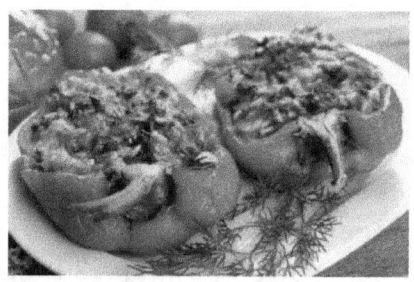

Time: 30 minutes

Serves: 4

Ingredients

4 ounces chorizo sausage, chopped
4 ounces lean ground beef
½ cup diced onion
¼ cup shredded low fat cheddar cheese
3 large eggs, beaten
2 medium red bell peppers

Directions
1. Preheat oven to 400°F. Line a baking sheet with foil.
2. Cook chorizo in a skillet until almost crispy. Drain excess fat and chop into small bits.
3. Place chorizo and ground beef in mixing bowl and combine with the onion, cheese and eggs.
4. Cut peppers in half lengthwise. Hollow out by removing seeds and cutting away ribs.
5. Fill each pepper with one-quarter of the meat mixture. Place on the prepared baking sheet. Bake for 25 to 30 minutes and serve hot.
6. Serve as an entrée or a side dish.

Nutritional Information

Serving Size: 175g, Calories: 239, Calories from Fat: 128, Total Fat: 14.2g, Saturated Fat: 4.7g, Trans Fat: 0.1g, Cholesterol: 190mg, Sodium: 329mg, Potassium: 399mg, Total Carbs: 5.3g, Dietary Fiber: 1.6g, Sugars: 3.5g, Protein: 21.2g

Salmon-Asparagus Crepes

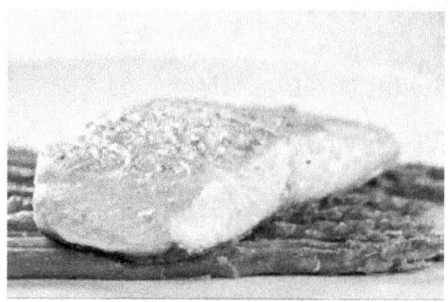

Time: 1 hour 30 minutes

Serves: 6

Ingredients

3 large eggs
2 tablespoons gluten free All Purpose Low-Carb Baking Mix
2 teaspoons extra virgin olive oil
1 tablespoon fat free half and half
2 teaspoons unsalted butter, divided in two portions
1 lemon
6 cups water
1 ½ teaspoons salt
1 teaspoon peppercorns
1 pound salmon fillet
1 pound asparagus, trimmed and cut into ¾-inch pieces
2 cups low fat Swiss cheese sauce

Directions

1. For crepe batter: In a blender, combine eggs, baking mix, half and half and one tablespoon water. Blend on high speed until batter is thin and smooth. To make crepes: Melt ¼ teaspoon of the butter in an eight-inch non-stick skillet over medium-high heat, add two tablespoons batter and swirl pan to coat bottom. Cook until lightly browned on the bottom, about one minute. Flip crepe with a spatula and cook until lightly browned (about 30 seconds). Transfer to a plate. Repeat with remaining batter (makes 8 crepes). Melt butter in skillet before each crepe.
2. For filling: Cut lemon in half; squeeze juice into a large skillet or shallow saucepan. Add water, salt and peppercorns and bring to a boil. Reduce heat to medium-low.
3. Add salmon and simmer until cooked through, about 10 minutes. Transfer salmon to a plate; flake with a fork, and remove any dark flakes underneath.
4. Heat oven to 375°F. Butter a 9- by 13-inch baking dish with two teaspoons butter.
5. Pour olive oil into a non-stick skillet over medium heat. Add asparagus and season with salt and pepper; cook until slightly tender, yet still crunchy, six to eight minutes.
6. Add one cup of the cheese sauce to asparagus and bring to a boil. Remove from heat and gently stir in the salmon. Let cool for five minutes.
7. Set crepes on a flat surface. Spoon **1/3** cup salmon mixture on each crepe and roll up; set, seam-side down, in baking dish. Cover top of crepes with remaining sauce and bake

until sauce is bubbling and edges are lightly browned, 25 to 30 minutes. Serve piping hot!

Nutritional Information

Serving Size: 439g, Calories: 197, Calories from Fat: 95, Total Fat: 10.6g, Saturated Fat: 3.3g, Trans Fat: 0g, Cholesterol: 133mg, Sodium: 568mg, Potassium: 497mg, Total Carbs: 7.4g, Dietary Fiber: 2.2g, Sugars: 2g, Protein: 19.8g

Pancetta N' Cabbage

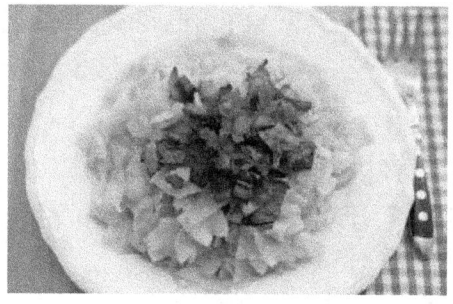

Time: 45 minutes

Serves: 4

Ingredients

1 ½ ounces pancetta, finely chopped
1 tablespoon extra virgin olive oil

½ cup finely chopped onion
½ cup finely chopped fennel bulb
4 cups thinly sliced green cabbage
¼ cup low sodium chicken broth
¼ teaspoon salt
¼ teaspoon crushed red pepper flakes
1 teaspoon white wine vinegar

Directions

1. Cook pancetta in a large skillet over medium-high heat, three to four minutes, until crisp. Transfer to a plate.
2. Add oil, onion and fennel to skillet and cook three minutes, until lightly caramelized. Add cabbage, broth, salt and crushed red pepper.
3. Reduce heat to medium; cover and cook until tender, 18 to 20 minutes.
4. Stir in white wine vinegar and pancetta.

Nutritional Information

Serving Size: 130g, Calories: 98, Calories from Fat: 64, Total Fat: 7.1g, Saturated Fat: 1.8g, Trans Fat: 0g, Cholesterol: 10mg, Sodium: 288mg, Potassium: 187mg, Total Carbs: 6.3g, Dietary Fiber: 2.4g, Sugars: 2.9g, Protein: 3.5g

Low Cal Indian Tikka Chicken

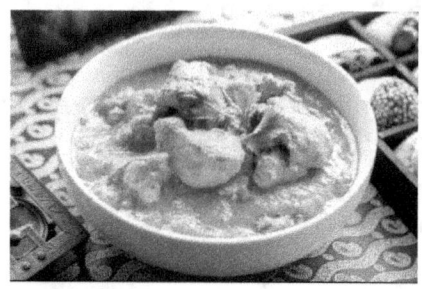

Time: 4 hours 30 minutes

Serves: 4

Ingredients

¾ cup Greek yogurt
1 tablespoon minced fresh ginger root
1 tablespoon chopped cilantro plus additional, for garnish
2 teaspoons chili powder
1 teaspoon ground coriander
1 teaspoon dried mint
1 tablespoon extra virgin olive oil
½ teaspoon salt
1 ½ pounds skinless, boneless chicken breasts cut into 1-inch cubes

Directions

1. Preheat oven to 375°F
2. In shallow bowl combine yogurt, ginger, cilantro, chili powder, coriander and mint and mix well. Mix the chicken cubes in the marinade and set in the refrigerator overnight for best results. Remove chicken from refrigerator and bring to room temperature approximately one hour before cooking.
3. Soak four to six thin wooden or bamboo skewers in water. Thread chicken on skewers, place on a baking sheet and drizzle with oil. Sprinkle with salt. Bake 30 minutes in the preheated oven, turning once halfway through cooking time, until golden brown and cooked through.
4. Sprinkle with chopped cilantro and garnish with lime.

Nutritional Information

Serving Size: 184g, Calories: 217, Calories from Fat: 79, Total Fat: 8.8g, Saturated Fat: 2.8g, Trans Fat: 0g, Cholesterol: 68mg, Sodium: 367mg, Potassium: 96mg, Total Carbs: 3.4g, Dietary Fiber: 0.7g, Sugars: 2.4g, Protein: 30.8g

Stuffed Turkey Breast With Arugula Salad

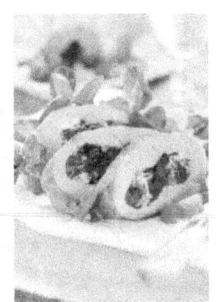

Time: 45 minutes

Serves: 4

Ingredients

2 tablespoons extra virgin olive oil
20 ounces frozen spinach, thaw and drain excess water
2/3 cup crumbled feta cheese
8 tablespoons ricotta cheese
8 green onions
2 tablespoons fresh chopped parsley
2 tablespoons fresh dill weed
2 large eggs
1 teaspoon salt
2/3 teaspoon black pepper
2/3 teaspoon garlic powder
2/3 teaspoon dried thyme
24 ounces turkey breast cutlet, pounded thin
8 cups arugula
20 cherry tomatoes
1 **2/3** cup canned lentils

Directions

1. Heat oven to 350°F.

2. Grease an eight-inch baking dish with half of the olive oil; set aside.
3. In a bowl, mix spinach, feta, ricotta, green onions, parsley, dill and egg until well combined. Spread a quarter of the spinach mixture down the center of each turkey cutlet.
4. Roll-up and place seam-side down in prepared baking dish. Hold together with a toothpick. Brush turkey roll with remaining olive oil. Sprinkle with salt, pepper, garlic powder and thyme. Bake about 30 minutes, until turkey is cooked through and stuffing is hot.
5. Combine arugula, tomatoes, lentils and dressing. Serve with turkey.

Nutritional Information

Serving Size: 1272g, Calories: 775, Calories from Fat: 303, Total Fat: 33.7g, Saturated Fat: 9.4g, Trans Fat: 0g, Cholesterol: 203mg, Sodium: 1593mg, Potassium: 2918mg, Total Carbs: 57.8g, Dietary Fiber: 16.3g, Sugars: 27g, Protein: 69.6g

Zucchini Pancakes With Feta, Walnuts And Oregano

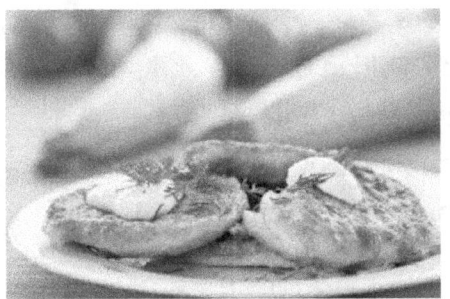

Time: 55 minutes

Serves: 5

Ingredients

2 medium zucchinis, trimmed and coarsely grated
½ teaspoon salt
3 green onions, chopped
3 large eggs, beaten
½ cup gluten-free All Purpose Low-Carb Baking Mix
1/3 cup fresh parsley, chopped
½ teaspoon ground pepper
3 ounces crumbled feta cheese
1/3 cup finely chopped walnuts
3 tablespoons olive oil

Directions

Toss zucchini with salt in a colander. Press zucchini with the back of a spoon and then blot between paper towels. Place in a medium bowl.

Add green onions, eggs, baking mix, parsley, oregano, and pepper; mix well. Fold in the feta and nuts. Turn oven to a warm setting (approximately 125°F)

Heat a non-stick skillet over medium-high heat and brush with oil. For each pancake, use one heaping tablespoon, and spread flat in pan, making four pancakes at a time, cooking about three minutes per side, until golden brown.

Keep finished pancakes warm in the oven until all the remaining batter has been used.

Nutritional Information

Serving Size: 169g, Calories: 268, Calories from Fat: 182, Total Fat: 20.3g, Saturated Fat: 5g, Trans Fat: 0g, Cholesterol: 127mg, Sodium: 575mg, Potassium: 349mg, Total Carbs: 14.4g, Dietary Fiber: 3g, Sugars: 2.6g, Protein: 10g

Taco Salad

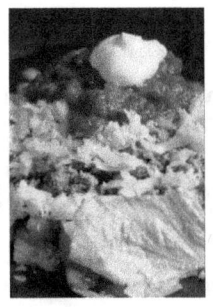

Time: 55 minutes

Serves: 4

Ingredients

1 tablespoon chili powder

1 teaspoon ground cumin
1 teaspoon gluten free Thicken Up (low carb food thickener)
½ teaspoon onion powder
½ teaspoon garlic powder
1 pound lean ground beef
¾ cup water
6 cups shredded Romaine lettuce
4 tablespoons taco sauce
4 ounces medium jicama (Mexican turnip), cut into thin strips
1 cup shredded fat free Monterey Jack cheese
½ cup shredded fat free cheddar cheese
4 tablespoons fat free sour cream

Directions

1. Make the seasoning mix: In a small bowl, combine the chili powder, cumin, Thicken Up, onion powder and garlic powder. Set aside.
2. In a large skillet, cook the ground beef over medium heat until browned, about 15 minutes.
3. Drain off fat, if any. Add the water and seasoning mix; stir to combine. Reduce heat to medium-low, and cook until liquid is almost completely absorbed, 10 to 12 minutes.
4. In a large bowl, toss lettuce with taco sauce. Divide among four large serving bowls, about 1 ½ cups each. Top each with ¼ cup chopped jicama.
5. In a medium bowl, toss the Monterey jack and cheddar cheeses together; divide and sprinkle over the jicama.

6. Spoon the beef mixture (about ½ cup per serving) over the cheese.
7. Top each with one tablespoon sour cream.

Nutritional Information

Serving Size: 311g, Calories: 293, Calories from Fat: 90, Total Fat: 10g, Saturated Fat: 4.2g, Trans Fat: 0g, Cholesterol: 109mg, Sodium: 719mg, Potassium: 668mg, Total Carbs: 11.1g, Dietary Fiber: 2.8g, Sugars: 3.7g, Protein: 37.9g

Shrimp Gumbo

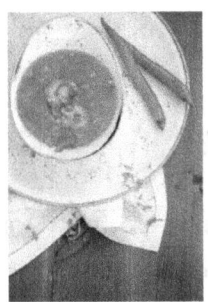

Time: 50 minutes

Serves: 6

Ingredients

3 tablespoons extra virgin olive oil, divided
2 tablespoons gluten free All Purpose Low-Carb Baking Mix

2 celery stalks, chopped
1 small green bell pepper, seeded and chopped
1 small onion, chopped
5 ½ cups chicken broth
1 cup diced stewed tomatoes
2 teaspoons Creole seasoning blend
2 tablespoons garlic cloves, chopped
1 pound collard greens, washed, cut in strips, or 2 packages (10-ounces each) frozen
1 (10-ounce) package frozen cut okra
2 pounds large shrimp, shelled and deveined

Directions

1. In a large saucepan, heat oil over medium heat, whisk in baking mix and cook, whisking, until deep golden brown, about five minutes.
2. Add celery, bell pepper and onion and cook 5 minutes, stirring occasionally, five minutes. Add garlic and creole seasoning and cook for one minute longer.
3. Add chicken broth and tomatoes to vegetable mixture and bring to a boil. Add collards and okra, cover and cook until collards are tender, about five minutes.
4. Add shrimp to gumbo, mix well, cover, and cook four minutes, until shrimp are pink and cooked through.
5. Season to taste with hot pepper sauce, salt and pepper.

Nutritional Information

Serving Size: 562g, Calories: 279, Calories from Fat: 81, Total Fat: 9g, Saturated Fat: 1.4g, Trans Fat: 0g, Cholesterol: 216mg, Sodium: 952mg, Potassium: 458mg, Total Carbs: 17g, Dietary Fiber: 5.2g, Sugars: 3.1g, Protein: 36.1g

Roast Beef And Mixed Greens With Pickled Okra And Radishes

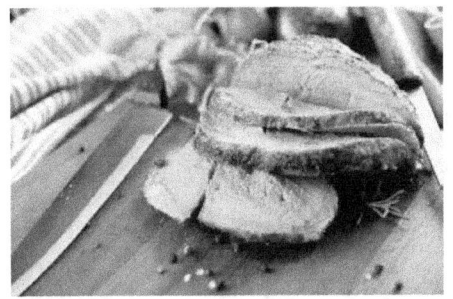

Time: 30 minutes

Serves: 8

Ingredients

48 ounces lean roast beef
8 cups mixed greens
16 ounces pickled okra
40 radishes, sliced
8 servings fat free Creamy Italian Dressing

Directions

1. Season roast beef with salt and freshly ground pepper.
2. Slice or cut beef into cubes, and serve cold or slightly warmed the microwave.
3. Toss greens, okra, and radishes with dressing. Serve salad with roast beef.

Nutritional Information

Serving Size: 531g, Calories: 385, Calories from Fat: 44, Total Fat: 4.8g, Saturated Fat: 1.6g, Trans Fat: 0g, Cholesterol: 122mg, Sodium: 2153mg, Potassium: 360mg, Total Carbs: 36.7g, Dietary Fiber: 9.4g, Sugars: 6.1g, Protein: 44.8g

Pork Tenderloin With Tomatoes And Green Olives

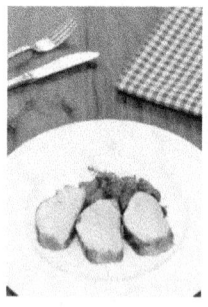

Time: 1 hour

Serves: 6

Ingredients

2 plum tomatoes, seeded and chopped
2 ounces chopped green olives
¼ cup dry white wine
1 teaspoon chopped fresh rosemary
2 garlic cloves, pushed through a press
1 tablespoon extra-virgin olive oil
1 ½ pounds whole pork tenderloins
½ teaspoon salt
¼ teaspoon ground pepper
1 cup low sodium chicken broth
2 teaspoons Thicken Up (food thickener)

Directions

1. Preheat oven to 400°F.
2. Combine tomatoes, olives, white wine, rosemary and garlic in a bowl.
3. Heat oil in a heavy ovenproof skillet over medium-high heat until hot. Season pork with salt and pepper. Sauté pork on both sides, about five minutes. Add tomato mixture.
4. Insert ovenproof meat thermometer into thickest part of pork. Place skillet in oven and bake 30 minutes, or until thermometer registers 160°F. Remove pork from skillet; cover and keep warm.

5. Place skillet over medium heat; add broth and Thicken Up. Bring to a boil; reduce heat and simmer until slightly thickened, five minutes. Drizzle sauce over pork and serve hot!

Nutritional Information

Serving Size: 181g, Calories: 159, Calories from Fat: 58, Total Fat: 6.4g, Saturated Fat: 1.8g, Trans Fat: 0g, Cholesterol: 43mg, Sodium: 786mg, Potassium: 101mg, Total Carbs: 8g, Dietary Fiber: 0.8g, Sugars: 3.1g, Protein: 15.1g

Pumpkin-Spice Brownies

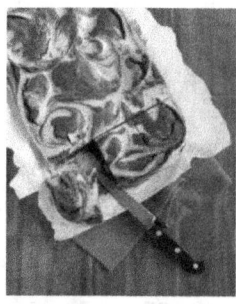

Time: 40 minutes

Serves: 16

Ingredients

2 ounces unsweetened baking chocolate
½ cup unsalted butter

1 tablespoon unsweetened cocoa powder

4 ounces powdered erythritol (sugar alcohol food additive)

4 large eggs

2 teaspoons vanilla extract

¼ cup coconut flour

¼ teaspoon baking soda

¼ teaspoon salt

½ teaspoon ground cinnamon

8 ounces fat free cream cheese

2/3 cup unsweetened pumpkin puree

1/3 cup granular sugar substitute (sucralose)

1 ½ teaspoons pumpkin pie spice

Directions

1. Preheat oven to 350°F.
2. Grease an 8x8-inch pan.
3. Melt butter and chocolate in a small bowl at 30-second intervals in the microwave until melted. Thoroughly mix the chocolate and butter together and add in the cocoa powder and powdered erythritol and continue to mix until smooth. Add one teaspoon vanilla and three eggs; whisk until incorporated. Whisk the coconut flour, baking soda, salt and cinnamon in a small bowl. Add to the chocolate mixture and stir until thickened. Set the brownie mixture aside.
4. Using a hand blender, mix the cream cheese with the sucralose in a small bowl. Add one egg, pumpkin purée, pumpkin spice blend and one teaspoon vanilla; beat until smooth.

5. Spread **2/3** of the brownie mixture into the prepared pan. Pour cream cheese mixture over the top. Drop the remaining **1/3** of the brownie batter by spoonfuls over the cream cheese mixture and then take a knife and gently swirl the layers together. Bake for 30 minutes. Allow to cool before cutting. Best served at room temperature but keep refrigerated in an airtight container for up to one week.

Nutritional Information

Serving Size: 56g, Calories: 142, Calories from Fat: 125, Total Fat: 13.9g, Saturated Fat: 8.3g, Trans Fat: 0g, Cholesterol: 77mg, Sodium: 156mg, Potassium: 72mg, Total Carbs: 9.8g, Dietary Fiber: 1.2g, Sugars: 7.7g, Protein: 3.4g

Spicy Turnip Fries

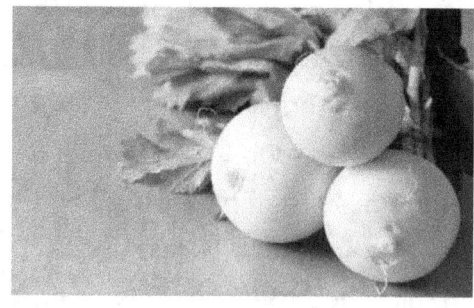

Time: 40 minutes

Serves: 6

Ingredients

4 turnips, trimmed and peeled (about 1 ¼ pounds)
2 tablespoons extra virgin olive oil
1 teaspoon Kosher salt
½ teaspoon chili powder

Directions

Heat oven to 425°F.
Cut turnips into 2½-inch sticks. Place on a foil-lined pan. Drizzle with oil and sprinkle with salt and chili powder. Toss with your hands to coat. Spread out in a single layer.
Bake fries 25 minutes, turning halfway through cooking time for even browning. Bake five more minutes under the broiler for extra crispy. Serve immediately.

Nutritional Information

Serving Size: 88g, Calories: 64, Calories from Fat: 42, Total Fat: 4.7g, Saturated Fat: 0.7g, Trans Fat: 0g, Cholesterol: 0mg, Sodium: 443mg, Potassium: 158mg, Total Carbs: 5.5g, Dietary Fiber: 1.4g, Sugars: 3.4g, Protein: 0.7g

Kale Chips

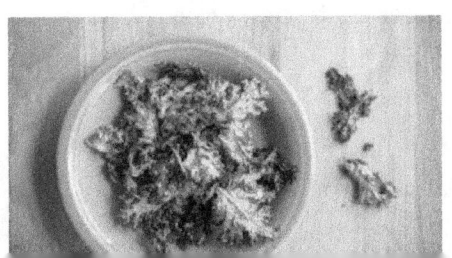

Time: 35 minutes

Serves: 6

Ingredients

7 ounces curly kale (trimmed from about 13 ounces, discard stems)
1 tablespoon extra-virgin olive oil
1/8 teaspoon sea salt

Directions

1. Preheat oven to 250°F and prepare a sheet pan with parchment paper.
2. Remove the leaves from the stems of the kale stalk. Tear leaves into bite-sized pieces.
3. Toss kale with olive oil by hand in a bowl then arrange equally spaced on the baking sheet and season with sea salt.
4. Place pan in the oven and set a timer for 30 minutes. After 20 minutes check to see if pieces are dried and crispy, if not continue to check at five minute intervals. Store in an airtight container up to one week.

Nutritional Information

Serving Size: 36g, Calories: 36, Calories from Fat: 21, Total Fat: 2.3g, Saturated Fat: 0g, Trans Fat: 0g, Cholesterol: 0mg, Sodium: 53mg, Potassium: 162mg, Total Carbs: 3.5g, Dietary Fiber: 0g, Sugars: 0g, Protein: 1g

Ham N' Cheese Frittata

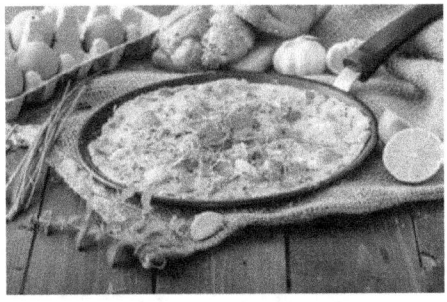

Time: 40 minutes

Serves: 6

Ingredients

1 tablespoon chopped yellow onion (½ small onion)
½ medium green bell pepper, chopped
8 ounces chopped cooked lean ham
3 tablespoons chopped Italian (flat leaf) parsley leaves, divided
9 large eggs, beaten

¼ cup half and half
¼ cup water
½ teaspoon salt
½ teaspoon Italian seasoning
1 cup grated fat free Swiss cheese, divided

Directions

1. Preheat broiler.
2. Melt butter in a large non-stick skillet over medium-high heat; add onion, pepper, ham and half the parsley. Cook five minutes, until onion is soft and translucent.
3. Combine eggs, half and half, water, salt, Italian seasoning and half the grated cheese.
4. Add egg mixture to pan. Cook, stirring constantly, until the eggs form soft, creamy curds, about five minutes. Remove from heat; sprinkle remaining cheese over top of eggs.
5. Place skillet under broiler; cook until cheese is bubbly and golden, about three minutes. Cool slightly.
6. Slide frittata onto a serving platter; top with remaining parsley.
7. Cut into wedges.

Nutritional Information

Serving Size: 164g, Calories: 166, Calories from Fat: 88, Total Fat: 9.8g, Saturated Fat: 3.3g, Trans Fat: 0g, Cholesterol: 300mg, Sodium: 705mg, Potassium: 393mg, Total Carbs: 2.2g, Dietary Fiber: 0g, Sugars: 1.1g, Protein: 17g

Roast Chicken And Vegetable Stew

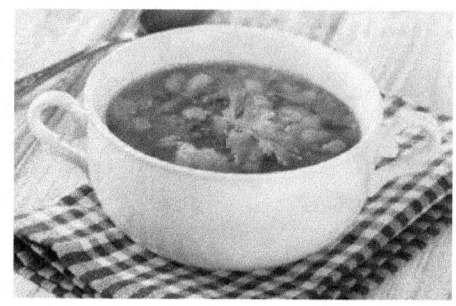

Time: 45 minutes

Serves: 6

Ingredients

2 ½ pounds roasted whole chicken
3 ½ cups low sodium chicken broth
1 bay leaf
2/3 cup half and half
3 tablespoons butter
¾ cup chopped red bell pepper
½ cup chopped white onion
½ pound fresh sliced mushrooms
17 ounces fresh asparagus spears, cut into 1-inch pieces
1 cup fresh green beans, cut into 1-inch pieces
1 tablespoon chopped fresh thyme
1/8 teaspoon salt

1/8 teaspoon ground black pepper

Directions

1. Remove chicken meat from the bones and skin. Cut into bite-sized pieces and place into a bowl and set aside.
2. Place half and half in a small saucepan and cook over medium heat until thick, five to seven minutes. While "cream" reduces, melt butter in a medium saucepan over high heat. Sauté bell pepper and onion until softened, about 3 minutes. Add broth and bay leaf and bring to a boil, about 10 minutes.
3. Add mushrooms, asparagus and green beans to the broth and cook until tender, about seven minutes. Add chicken and simmer on low until heated through, about three minutes.
4. Turn off heat and stir in reduced cream and thyme. Season to taste with salt and pepper.

Nutritional Information

Serving Size: 484g, Calories: 423, Calories from Fat: 261, Total Fat: 29g, Saturated Fat: 11.9g, Trans Fat: 0g, Cholesterol: 160mg, Sodium: 1031mg, Potassium: 402mg, Total Carbs: 11.4g, Dietary Fiber: 3.4g, Sugars: 5.2g, Protein: 34.4g

Coconut-Almond Cookies

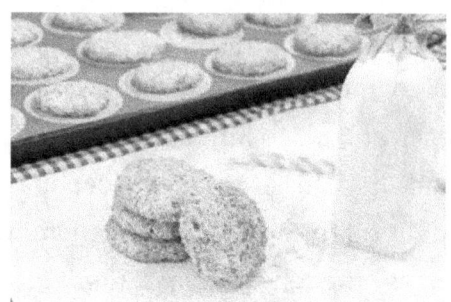

Time: 35 minutes

Serves: 12

Ingredients

Olive oil cooking spray to prepare pans
½ cup almond flour
1/3 cup unsweetened shredded coconut
2 ounces hazelnuts (about ¼ cup)
2 large egg whites
2 tablespoons seltzer water
1 ½ teaspoons coconut extract
1 teaspoon vanilla extract
½ teaspoon salt
8 tablespoons unsalted butter
7 tablespoons granular sugar substitute (sucralose)

Directions

Preheat oven to 350°F.

Toast hazelnuts in an even layer on a cookie sheet for eight minutes. Cool, coarsely chop and set aside.

Increase oven temperature to 375°F. Grease baking sheet with cooking spray.

In large bowl, combine almond flour, coconut, hazelnuts, egg whites, seltzer, coconut and vanilla extracts, salt, butter and sugar substitute. Mix well.

Drop by one tablespoon per cookie (makes 12) onto prepared baking sheet. Bake 20 minutes, or until light golden brown. Cool cookies on baking sheet one minute before transferring to wire racks to cool completely.

Nutritional Information

Serving Size: 42g, Calories: 107, Calories from Fat: 100, Total Fat: 11.1g, Saturated Fat: 5.1g, Trans Fat: 0g, Cholesterol: 20mg, Sodium: 161mg, Potassium: 51mg, Total Carbs: 1g, Dietary Fiber: 0.6g, Sugars: 0g, Protein: 1.6g

Camembert Cheese

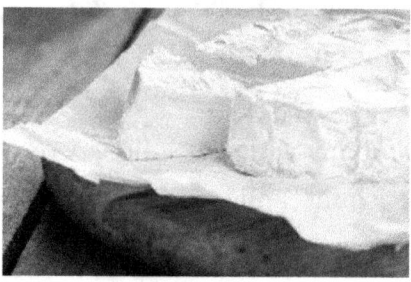

Camembert cheese is a cheese that comes from France and is made with milk. It's a softer cheese that looks great if you're looking to impress.

Ingredients

1 gallon fresh whole milk
1 ¼ pint cream
¼ teaspoon mesophilic cheese culture
1/8 teaspoon camemberti mold culture
1/8 teaspoon rennet
1 tbsp fine sea salt

Equipment

Large pan
Long knife

Cheese cloth

Dairy thermometer

Colander

Large bowl

Moulds or perforated straight sided pots or dishes

Directions

1. Heat the milk and cream together gently to 86ºF.
2. Sprinkle in the cheese culture and the camemberti culture
3. Leave to rest for 1 and a half hours.
4. Dilute the rennet according to the instructions and add to the cultured milk
5. Once the curds are firm slice into 1/2 inch cubes with the knife.
6. Using the colander in a large bowl line it with the cheese cloth and scoop the curds in. Leave to drain whey from the curds. Leave for an hour.
7. Remove the cheese from the colander and fill moulds. Leave for 24 hours then unmould.
8. Sprinkle the outside with salt
9. Stand cheeses in a constant temperature as far as possible at 45ºF for 8 weeks

Part 2

Introduction

Are you tired of the ever-increasing number on your scale?
Are you sick of the looks of judgment from your loved ones and strangers?
Do you only see yourself as a lump of unwanted fat instead of a human being?
Are you exhausted from researching and attempting new fad diets, only to be constantly disappointed with your results and decreasing budget?
Well, you have come to the right place! I congratulate you! If you came across this book, you are on the hunt for useful information on ways that you can transform your beautiful self into a person you can love each and every day instead of insulting your body!
If you have never heard of the Atkins Diet, you are in for a treat! Tucked away within the contents of this book:

- How to develop a healthy mindset to begin the journey of creating a better version of yourself
- How to stay motivated, even when you feel like giving up and fleeing to that bag of potato chips
- Why you should choose the Atkins Diet
- How the Atkins Diet actually works, in details that anyone can grasp
- Tips and tricks that can help you stay on track and avoid temptations while on the Atkins Diet train
- And more!

Isn't it about time that you started on the path to feel better about yourself, both inside and out?

Isn't it time that you find a diet plan that can REALLY work for you and your hectic lifestyle, without sacrificing your taste buds' happiness? We are human beings, not robots, so why should you give away your soul to the fakeness of fad dieting? That's right, you shouldn't! With the purchase of this book, you can unlock all the secrets you need to get on a diet plan that will work with you, not against you.

Because every diet starts with you, starts from you.

This is not just a dieting plan. This book holds the key to an entirely new lifestyle to get you on the right path to feeling great!

Why is this particular book different than the other dieting guides you have spent your hard-earned money on?

Two reasons:

1. It assumes that a diet is the whole lifestyle, not only meals. Then it requires your mindset and commitment.
2. It provides realistic tips and tricks to keep you from veering off your path to your goal weight. With the dawn of a new-fangled lifestyle comes the need for a positively sparkling mindset, to keep your head clear for those days that you just want to grab that forsaken cookie jar and give up entirely. No. You can do better, and this book is a perfect map to find your way to that pristine looking you!

Chapter 1: Every Diet Starts With You!

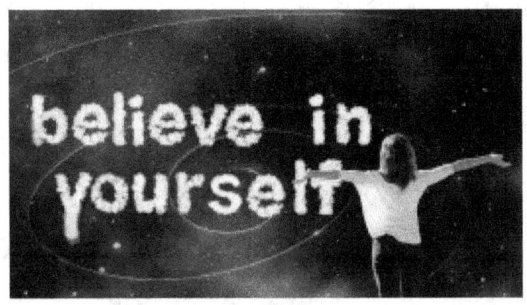

Each and every dieting strategy has its pros and cons, but before even engulfing yourself in the rulebook of whichever one you would like to try out, you must step into the right mindset, and learn how to truly live within its means. Many believe that "being on a mission to 'fix' themselves" is the perfect mindset to get down and dirty with a weight loss program. This is an entirely OPPOSITE psyche that one should be in when it comes to deciding to shed that extra weight they are tired of lugging around. This is a terrible way to think, due to the fact that people will lunge for the first diet plan that comes across their computer screens, and out of desperation they will try it. Then, they get absolutely obsessed with results. Naturally as human beings, our minds are hardwired to want instant gratification. Individuals who are on these "quick-losing fad diets" do not see the number on their scales dropping as fast as they would like, and give up, going back to their potato chip eating, couch potato ways in order to soothe their battered souls and mighty hunger pains.

Obviously, thinking and functioning this way is beyond destructive. Negative minds lead to paths of failure. This chapter is full of ways to kick start your way to having a more positive outlook of yourself and your body, and how you can not "fix it" but make the best better!

Focus on attainability – It is important to be realistic with your expectations. If you have not worked out in years, hitting the gym, lifting beyond your weight limit and running 30 minutes on an elliptical is going to quickly get you to a give-up point. Start with a more attainable goal, like a 20-30 minute walk. If you are not much of a chef and feel like you cannot maintain portion control as much as you should be, try out pre-packed delivery services, such as Blue Apron or HelloFresh, that have pre-portioned ingredients and detailed instructions. This will assist you in becoming familiar with healthy ingredients, and learn fundamental cooking skills that you can later use to make your own healthy and delicious meals.

Throw out the thoughts of "Foods are good or bad" – In our society, we have naturally learned that we should either feel great or ashamed by the choices we make when purchasing edibles to consume. You should not feel guilty for eating a sweet or two here and there. It is important to remember that all foods can fit in a diet.

Positively communicate with yourself – Would you tell your friend that they look terrible or look fat in what they are wearing? Probably not. You should use the same mentality when giving yourself a pep-talk in front of the mirror. In this day and age, we are unbelievably difficult on ourselves, thanks to society's standards of beauty and image. Practice positive communication with yourself, instead of beating yourself up.

Put your scale away – Scales are not totally bad guys, but they are used way too often when it comes to terms of losing weight. They are used as negative tools when it comes to our weight loss goals, and instant gratification. They lead only to destructive thoughts. It is pretty crucial to get to a mindset and a point into your weight loss journey before stepping upon a scale. The number that it displays does not define your worth.

Truly know your "troubled thoughts" – If you know that you binge eat ice cream when you are stressed, make a mental note of it. If you are constantly bashing yourself when in front of the mirror, remember that. During this step, it is of good practice to consciously say "stop!" to yourself out loud. This action is all it takes for some to break the cycle of bad habits. This also allows room for you to make much healthier decisions.

Take down the calendar –

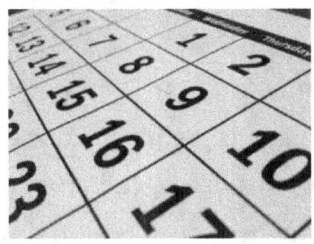

Patience is a virtue, and one that many of us do not know how to put into action, especially when it comes to our weight loss journeys. If you make more attainable goals, such as walking 10,000 steps a day, every day, there is no room to have your mind wrapped around the idea of a "deadline" to achieve your goals. Each day is full of new possibilities. Reach for the sky every day and you will start to see major progress!

Learn to take a breath or two

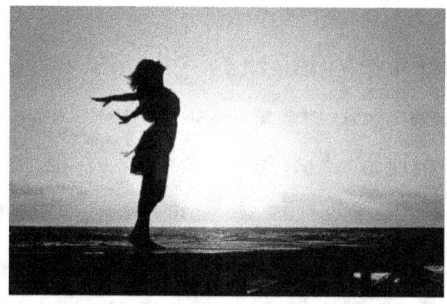

– Spend some time before you start your day or before you begin your workout to focus on simply breathing. This helps you become deeply connected with your body, lower stress responses and sets your intentions for yourself. Sounds silly, but it really works!

Reinvent rewards and punishments – You have to truly believe that making healthier choices is helping you pave the path for better self-care. Food should not be considered a reward, and exercise should not be thought of as a type of punishment. They both go hand in hand when taking care of you and your body. Viewing your body as a temple instead of a body image issue is a great way to get into the proper mindset.

Greet positivity with open arms –

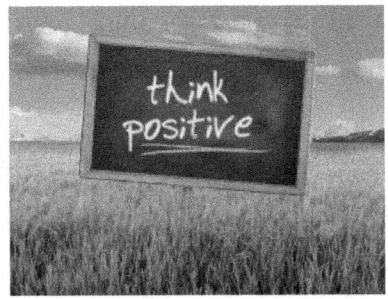

Surround yourself with positive individuals. This will give you an encouraging support system, and will constantly remind you of your health goals. Engulfing yourself with positivity, inside and out, is the perfect fuel to provide you with the momentum to keep going forward even when you feel like giving up.

Change up your goals – The result should be to lose your unwanted weight, but it should not be your actual goal. Goals should be sustainable things that you have full control over. Did you catch 8 hours of sleep? There's a great goal for your health met. Did you consume 5 servings of vegetables and fruits? If not, you now know what direction to go in for the remainder of your day. Do not beat yourself up if you do not achieve all your small health goals for the day. We are human, after all.

Chapter 2: Why The Atkins Diet?

When many hear the word "diet", they just think of one thing: losing weight. But it really has two meaning. Yes, shedding unwanted weight and getting yourself to a healthier point is one. But "diet" shouldn't put a bad taste in our mouth (literally). It is a permanent and fundamental part of all our lifestyles, no matter what they may be. Your daily diet should be something that enriches your life, not weighs you down (no pun intended). Many individuals go into the world of shedding their excess pounds with a short-term way of thinking about what they are consuming and how fast the number on the scale should diminish. To be truly successful when changing anything about your diet in terms of what you consume, one should look at a diet as an everyday task of eating and drinking regularly. It is WHAT you eat and drink that matters. And no, one should not have to waste away their days consuming cardboard-like foods, either.

So, why choose the Atkins diet to incorporate into your daily routine? Great question! The Atkins Diet was actually first introduced clear back in 1972 by Dr. Robert Atkins. The original plan restricted the act of consuming foods that had high carbohydrate counts, such as bread, rice, pastas and starchy veggies. Atkins advocated the idea that carbs increased blood sugar levels that released insulin, which helps prevent fat from breaking down and being absorbed into our bodies.

Since the 1970's, the theory of the Atkins Diet still holds true. It works around the notion that gains in weight is caused by the way our bodies handle the breakdown of those pesky carbohydrates. As you can imagine, this diet has been one of the most controversial, yet, it has remained one of the most popular diet brands known today.

So, why should you choose it? Here is why!

Lose weight and still eat your favorites – Within the majority of diets lies the restriction of eating high in fat foods such as cream, butter, bacon and steak, just to name a few. In fact, they are pretty forbidden items to consume on almost all diets. But not on the Atkins! They are actually encouraged here.

Hunger pains are a thing of the past – For those that have battled their way through virtually impossible to live off of diets, the Atkins is much different. As long as one sticks close to the "permitted" foods, there is actually no set limit to how much you can actually eat. Throwing out foods that have a high number of carbohydrates keeps your blood sugars at a stable level, which means your tummy won't be rumbling in-between meals.

Fast results – For those that follow the way of the Atkins diet closely and by the rules will see compelling weight loss, especially during the most restrictive phases you go through when you begin the Atkins diet, which we will get to later. Like we have discussed before, everyone enjoys instant gratification, and this keeps those on this diet motivated if they see physical changes, as well as a lowered number upon the scale.

Results stick around – The Atkins diet not only produces fast results, but creates results that stick around! The secret is that this diet is not one that you have to abide by the rules of a low-calorie or a low-fat diet, but this is a low-CARB diet. So, more individuals will want to abide by the Atkins rulebook than those of other diets, which leave them fatigued and feeling pretty gloomy about their appearance.

Lower health risks – The Atkins diet, unlike most, encourages individuals to consume foods high in protein. Instead of a feeling of light-headiness and constant hunger pains, one feels fuller and ready to conquer the day. It also recommends only certain fruits and veggies, enough to keep your digestive track up to par as your venture into the Atkins.

It is a proven diet – Most diets on the market having more warning labels when going to purchase than they do positive labels, which, in itself, should veer many consumers away. But the desperation to lose weight makes many dismiss the warning labels and put their bodies through mayhem.

Not time-consuming or expensive – Those that are in the diet company business know exactly what to say to say to attract their most potential customers, which typically involves consumers spending quite a chunk of their hard-earned cash to participate in diets that spill out a bunch of false promises but give nothing but disappointments. Also, many other diets are quite time-consuming, from spending money on nifty little containers to put portions of edibles in, to chopping up food for portion control, to spending time and money at the grocery store picking out the "proper foods" that fit within the diet's restrictions…it is a chaotic waste of valuable time.

Convenience – Building your own healthy meal at home can take up time, as stated above. The Atkins diet actually launched a frozen-foods line back in 2013, which was named the very first low-carb frozen-food line on the market that is available for any consumers to buy and combine into their regular diets. Atkins also offers convenience foods, likes shakes, snack bars and baking mixes to use.

Varieties of delicious recipes – Atkins not only provides detailed meal plans with options to choose from, but also has a broad variety of recipes that one can make at home, with ingredients and carb counts included. Included later in this book are Atkins Diet approved recipes for all parts of your day!

Ability to still eat out – Unlike many diets that prohibit you from enjoying a night out on the town with a loved one or friends, Atkins actually has a list of approved fast food places, as well as specific restaurant options, depending on what phase you are on within the Atkins diet at the time. If you are not shy and like asking questions about what is in your meal, ask away! You will feel better about what you are shoveling into your temple in the first place this way too.

Lots of cool extras – The Atkins diet comes equipped with a free meal planner as well as a two-week meal plan, a carb counter and forums that you can communicate with others on their Atkins journey. You are by no means alone!

Amazing tastes – On the Atkins, the diet does not prohibit you from eating some of your flavorful favorites. What is not to like about a juicy steak or a meaty cheeseburger? Many diets would make you eat the meat without a bun, and that is just no fun!

Of course, there are some cons to each and every diet plan known to man. But, we will not venture into that here. As you can see, from the pros listed above, there are many reasons as to why you should choose the Atkins diet as your first diet plan to venture into, or make it your last one if you are an individual who has battled with countless plans that leaves nothing but disappointment in yourself, empty stomachs and even emptier pockets.

Chapter 3: How The Atkins Diet Works

Atkins is a pretty well-known name throughout a variety of cultures. But what many don't know is that the Atkins Diet has helped millions of individuals lose weight, and has been doing so for over 20 years. Dr. Atkins hit the knowledge lottery with this one, as he has referred to this diet as "ongoing weight loss."

The question you probably have at this point now is, "How in the world does a diet such as this WORK?" And "how can I make is work well for me?"

The Atkins Diet is made up of four differently unique phases that dieters partake in. Each phase involves very little carbohydrate intake and focuses on eating more over time until you achieve you desired weight. Sounds a bit confusing and counteractive, I know. But one has to remember one of the main rules of Atkins. Pushing carbs away from you is not quite as simple as telling sugar to back off. You must stick to the list of acceptable to eat foods, as well as get in touch with your arithmetic skills. For example, within Phase 1 you are allowed 20 grams of "net carbs" per day, with 12-15 of those being from the "foundation veggies" on your list. But, the best part? You do not have to trim off the fat off that tender and juicy steak if you do not wish to!

So, now that you have had a bit of a taste as to what the Atkins Diet is and inkling into the way it functions to assist you in your weight loss journey, lets dig right in the entrée of the Atkins Diet to see how it works and how it can work for you!

Phase 1: Induction

First things first, this phase is not for everyone. Here is a rough guide into making sure that taking the beginning steps within this phase is right for you:

- ✓ You want to lose a bit of weight QUICKLY
- ✓ You have unfortunately regained all the weight you managed to lose previously
- ✓ You have a slow/slowed down metabolism or are rather inactive
- ✓ You goal weight to shed is 14 pounds or higher

If you fall into any of those categories, let's step right into Phase 1! This phase is all about the transformation of your body. You want it to be a fat burning machine! Induction is all about limiting the amount of carbohydrates you consume, which you will be limited to about 20 grams of carbs per day. This is going to kick start your body into switching what its main source of fuel is, from carbs to fat.

Phase 1's goal is to help you decipher the difference between hunger from habit, and changing the foods you consume to better suit your appetite as it decreases. When you feel hungry, eat until you have satisfied that hunger but are not so full that you cannot function properly. It is important to remember to be patient, and wait roughly 10 or so minutes before you grab yourself something else to eat. Drink a glass of water instead. Instead of skipping meals when you are not hungry, grab a nice low in carb snack!

Phase 1 Guidelines

- Drink 8 glass of water (or other adequate drinks that are allowed) per day
- Eat 3 regular sized meals or 4-5 smaller meals per day
- Do NOT skip over meals or go any longer than 6 hours per day without eating
- For every meal, eat foods that are rich in proteins, at least 115-175 grams per meal
- Eat around 20 grams of carbohydrates per day
  o 12-15 of your carb intake should be from cooked veggies or salad
- You are allowed to take a multivitamin tablet and an omega-3 fatty acid supplement to ensure your body is receiving the nutrients it needs to function properly.

Phase 2: Ongoing Weight Loss

Now that you got a hang for the low-carb lifestyle, you can now consume a greater variety of different eats! Phase 2 is about finding your tolerance for low carb, in other words, the level of carbohydrates you can consume on a daily basis while you continue to steadily shed pounds at a good rate. Phase 2 is a right fit for you if:

✓ You are a vegetarian
✓ You have more weight you wish to shed but want to enjoy a bigger variety of food
✓ You are content with shedding pounds at a slower rate
✓ Your goal is to lose less than 14 pounds

If you only have a few pounds that you wish to shed or you live a vegetarian lifestyle, you can skip Phase 1 and step into the grips of Phase 2. Within this phase, you are to increase your intake of carbs bit by bit until you find your balance and tolerance. You are now allowed certain types of cheeses, berries, seeds and nuts, as well as Atkins food products.

Phase 2 Guidelines

Drink 8 glasses of water (or other allowed drinks) per day

Continue to take your multivitamin or other supplements if you decided to take them

Eat lots of foods with natural fats

Ensure that you are keeping track of the carbs you intake, which is easy to do with the Atkins carb counter

You can consume Atkins food products

You can consume an extra 5 grams of carbs per week, as you find your carb tolerance and balance

Unlike popular belief, steady weight loss happens more within this phase than in Phase 1, so be patient with yourself. Stick to the rules and you will eventually obtain your weight goal!

By increasing your intake of carbohydrates, you will eventually find out just how many carbs you can consume while still working toward you weight loss goal. This will help you form a healthier foundation in the long run, which will help you continuously stick close to your low carb lifestyle for life!

Phase 3: Pre-Maintenance

As you begin to see the light at the end of the tunnel with your weight loss goal, Phase 3 is about assisting in the establishment of healthier and long-term way of consuming foods the enrich your body, so that you can continue to stay happy and healthy for the long haul! Just like when hitting a target, slow and steady wins the race. During Phase 3 you are continuing to build up your carb tolerance so that when it is your time to enter the means of Phase 4, you know what works for YOU and your body long term. Nobody's body is quite the same, so what works for one person will more than likely not work exactly the same for the next. It is crucial that you listen to what your body is informing you of. During Phase 3, you are to increase your carb intake by 10 grams per week, so that you can find the right balance that works well for you! This phase is a lot about trial and error, so it is important to take your time, work at your own pace and listen to your physical well-being.

By the time you manage to reach your goal weight (YAY) you will know for sure what carbs your body can handle, and which ones you are better off avoiding. A major part of Phase 3 is about fine-tuning your carbs. If you have cravings that start to haunt and take a hold or you, or if that number on the scale starts to creep back up instead of staying down, decrease your carb intake by 10 grams per week, then re-introduce 5 grams back into your diet until you find your unique level that you can handle. Balance is everything, and you will find your perfect balance within Phase 3.
Keep in mind that the pounds will start to shed slower as you work on finding your carbohydrate balance. Patience is key!
Phase 3 Guidelines
- Drink 8 glasses of water (or other allowed beverage) per day
- Ensure that you monitor your intake of daily carbs, which assistance from the carb counter
- You are allowed to add grains, more fruits, starchy veggies into your diet

- You are allowed to add 10 grams of carbs per week as you find your carb balance

Phase 4: Maintenance

If you have made it to the fourth and final phase, congrats! By now you have managed to do what you thought before was impossible, which is reach and maintain your goal weight! Do not take this achievement lightly, for this is one of the main struggles that all adults face throughout their lifetime. Phase 4 is about keeping up the good work, and learning how to truly enjoy the low carb lifestyle! You are now aware of the do's and don'ts of your body, which foods work best and which edibles to avoid consuming. But that does not mean the works stops here for you! Diet changes are lifestyle changes. If you continue to stick beside the carb balance that you have refined for yourself over the past couple months, there is very little that can stop you from maintaining and keeping you looking and feeling sexy!

We are all human, and we make mistakes and have major slip ups. But do not start to panic if you start to gain a pound or two or more. One of the superb things about the Atkins diet is that you can get right back on it by simply dropping your carb intake by about 10-20 grams per week to regain control and continue your momentum!

You can continue to consume and enjoy the same varieties of foods that you ate during Phase 3, **as long as you are ensuring that you fat intake decreases as your carb intake increases.** Also, being an active individual is a big part of maintaining the new you that you are now proud to flaunt around. If you are not exercising, ensure that you start getting up and moving around!

It is a great way to keep the weight off, among the hundreds of other health benefits you receive from getting and remaining active every day!

Foods to Avoid while on the Atkins Diet
- **Legumes** – lentils, chickpeas, beans, etc (to be avoided during induction only)
- **Starches** – Potatoes, sweet potatoes (to be avoided during induction only)
- **High-carb fruits** – Grapes, pears, bananas, apples, oranges (induction only)
- **High-carb veggies** – Turnips, carrots, etc. (induction only)
- **Diet and low-fat foods** – Typically very high in sugar
- **Trans fats** – These are typically located in processed foods, look for the word "hydrogenated" within a foods' list of ingredients.
- **Vegetable oils** – Canola oil, cottonseed oil, corn oil, soybean oil, amongst others.
- **Grains** – Rice, barley, spelt, rye, wheat, etc.
- **Sugar** – (OBVIOUSLY) ice cream, candy, cakes, juices, soft drinks, etc.

Foods to Consume while on the Atkins Diet

- **Healthy fats** – Avocado oil, avocados, coconut oil, extra virgin olive oil, etc.
- **Nuts and seeds** – Sunflower seeds, walnuts, macadamia nuts, almonds, etc.
- **Full-fat dairy** – Full-fat yogurt, cream, cheese, butter, etc.

- **Low-carb veggies** – asparagus, broccoli, spinach, kale, etc.
- **Eggs** – eggs are known for their richness in Omega-3's
- **Fatty fish and seafood** – sardines, trout, salmon, etc.
- **Meats** – bacon, chicken, lamb, pork, beef, etc.
- **Acceptable drinks** – water, coffee, green tea

One Week Menu For Atkins

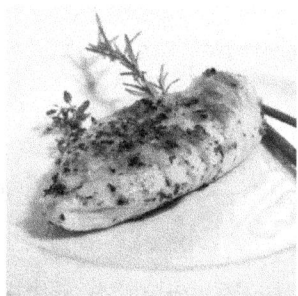

Below is a sample menu for those that are just starting out on the Atkins Diet but are unsure where to turn next. This week-long menu is best suited for those that are undergoing the induction phase. But you can use this menu as a base for those other phases, just be sure that you are slowly adding in veggies and fruits that are higher in carb counts as you continue forth.

Monday

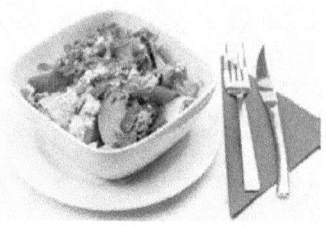

- Breakfast – Veggies and eggs, fried up on coconut oil
- Lunch – Chicken salad with olive oil, topped with a handful of nuts
- Dinner – Steak and veggies

Tuesday

- Breakfast – Eggs and bacon
- Lunch – Leftover chicken and veggies from the evening before
- Dinner – Cheeseburger minus the bun with veggies and butter

Wednesday

- Breakfast – An omelet with veggies, fried up in butter
- Lunch – Shrimp salad with olive oil
- Dinner – Ground beef stir fry paired with veggies

Thursday

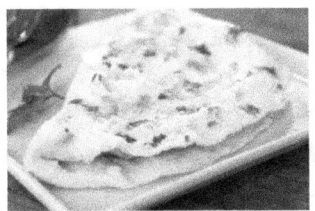

- Breakfast – Veggies with eggs, friend in coconut oil
- Lunch – Leftovers of the stir fry from the night before
- Dinner – Salmon with a pad of butter, paired with veggies

Friday

- Breakfast – Bacon and eggs
- Lunch – Chicken salad with olive oil, topped with a handful of nuts
- Dinner – Meatballs paired with veggies

Saturday

- Breakfast – Veggie omelet, fried up in butter
- Lunch – Leftover meatballs from night before
- Dinner – Pork chops paired with veggies

Sunday

- Breakfast – Eggs and bacon
- Lunch – Leftover pork chops from the night before
- Dinner – Grilled chicken wings, paired with veggies and salsa

Healthy Low-Carb Snacks

Many people who have picked and stuck with the Atkins diet have reported that their appetite actually decreases, and they tend to only eat 2 full meals per day instead of 3. Now, not everyone's diet or appetite is quite the same. If you feel hungry in-between meals, eat one of the below healthy, low-carb snacks to keep your tummy satisfied until further ado!

- Fruits (can eat after induction)
- Baby carrots (can eat in moderation during induction)
- Berries and whipped cream
- Greek yogurt
- Handful of nuts
- A portioned piece of meat
- Portioned cheese
- 1-2 hard boiled eggs
- Leftovers

Chapter 4: Tips And Tricks To Be Successful While On The Atkins Diet

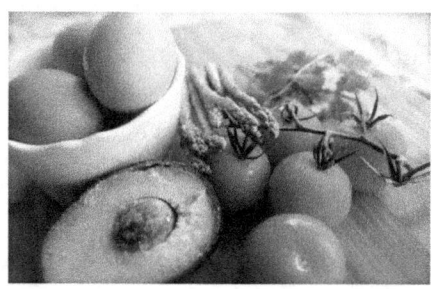

There is a lot of room to move around when on the Atkins Diet. While there are some key restrictions, they are something almost every individual can end up working with, which is a big reason that it has worked for so many people for the last couple decades. But, just like when beginning any new diet or lifestyle change, there is also room to revert back to your bad habits and terrible ways of eating. Another great aspect of the Atkins Diet is if you do an amazing job at sticking to the basic rulebook during the Induction Phase, you are unknowingly building a strong foundation to stand upon as you move forward into the other three phases of the diet. and narrow during the Induction Phase, which is also the most crucial for your success on the Atkins Diet.

Take a peek in your medicine cabinet – Sounds strange, but there are certain over the counter medicines that can slow your weight loss way down. Among these are non-steroidal anti-inflammatory drugs. These pain relievers tend to cause water retention and may actually block your body's ability to burn fat at the rate the Atkins Diet wishes you to do so. Cut back as much as you can, without risking injury or suffering, of course. If you need additional pain relief, try non-steroidal products. Obviously this as general rule of thumb. In each case, ask first your physician.

Keep track of your weight and measurements – While it is not healthy to step upon the dreaded scale multiple times a week or many times a day, weighing yourself is an important part in keeping track of your weight loss progress. Make a habit to record your weight on the first day of each month. You can weigh yourself more often, but ensure that you are actually writing the number upon your scale monthly. Recording weight on a daily basis can leave one feeling defeated, for one's weight will fluctuate some throughout the month. This is the same for your body measurements. When you are just beginning the Atkins diet, make sure to write down your measurements, and record them on the same day you write down your monthly weight. The numbers of your measurements can motivate you more so than the number of the scale!

Keep track of calories – A wonderful thing about the Atkins Diet is that you are not required to keep track of all those pesky calories. However, you still must watch what you are consuming. It is no secret that too much of a good thing can majorly contribute to packing on excess pounds. It is important to stick to a range of calories per day, 1,500-1,800 for women and 1,800-2,200 for men. It is time to cut back on those calories if you do not seem to be losing much or any weight.

Get out the pencil and paper – A popular habit that many of those on the mission to lose weight is the keeping of a well-documented and detailed food journal. Record what you eat during the day, what times you consume particular items etc. This allows one to see their eating habits that they may not realize otherwise. It is also a good method when you are attempting to count calories.

Beware of carbs in hiding – If you are unsure about certain foods, take the time to read the product label and search through the nutrition facts as well as the ingredient lists. You can avoid those excess sugars that lead to a build up of carbs later on. Just because a pretty package says what's inside is low in calories does not mean it is low-carb. Avoid these at all costs, unless the packaging is specifically labeled "low-carb". It is also important to use full-fat versions of foods, such as mayo, dressings etc. Low-fat versions add in extra sugar to assist with flavor replacement.

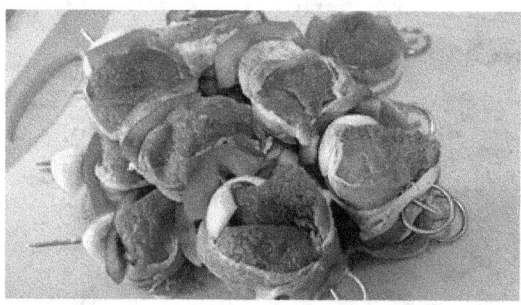

Eat enough to satisfy your tummy's needs – In order to kick start your body to start burning fat; you must consume enough dietary fat. Natural fats are great sources to consume if you learn to control your intake of carbs. But do not fall into the assumption that you are allowed to eat as much fat as you want. Fat calories can add up just as quickly if you let them.

Consume 4-6 ounces of protein PER meal – The amount of protein that you should eat every meal greatly depends on your body chemistry, especially gender and height. A woman that is on the petite side may be perfectly satisfied with consuming 4 ounces, as the guy next to her actually needs 6 ounces to be fully satisfied. Protein is a BIG factor in the terms of weight loss. Eating too much protein, not enough or eating just protein can interfere greatly with your weight loss results, as well as make you feel hungry, which leaves you susceptible to getting carb cravings.

Skimp on the salt – Your body needs salt, but many foods nowadays contain a great excess of the mineral. Too much salt can lead to weakness, headaches, muscle cramps and lightheadedness. Thankfully, Atkins diet is a diuretic diet, so you don't really need to avoid salt to help minimize your water retention levels.

Drink plenty of water and other fluids – It is recommended that all of us should be consuming at least 8 glasses of water or other fluids per day, and for some individuals they need more! Your urine can tell your story of how much fluids you are consuming. People should always try to aim for clear or pale urine. Never skip fluid intake so that you can see a lower number on your scale. It is counteractive. And in actuality, skimping on fluids can actually cause your body to retain fluid as a way to protect your body from becoming dehydrated.

Eat those veggies – You should be consuming at least 12-15 grams of your net carbs in the form of vegetables. Constipation can result from not eating enough fiber, which can make quite an impact on your scale number. The fiber hidden in veggies also assists in that full stomach feeling, which we all would like to have more often. Satisfying your hunger is big problem when it comes to implementing a diet and actually sticking to it.

Avoid sweeteners – Most sweeteners claim to be 0 carb and contain 0 calories, but they still cause excessive weight gain. It does not matter the brand that you purchase, all artificial sweeteners are all one in the same. They only spike your blood sugar level, which tells your body to store extra insulin, leading to the packing on of excess fat. This includes products that artificial sweeteners are in as well, like diet soda, crystal light, tonic water, chewing gum and sugar-free Jell-O, just to name a few. You are limited to 3 servings of fake sweeteners each day while on the Atkins diet. Obviously, the less you consume the better.

Ensure you are keeping track of net carbs – While on the Atkins Diet, you need to ensure that you are really getting the most out of your allowed 20 grams of net carbs per day. Condiments such as lemon juice should be counted as at least 1 net carb, especially condiments like ketchup, which contain quite a bit of sugar. Try your best to not utilize your carb allowance for edibles that are initially high in starches and other sugar, and low in fiber.

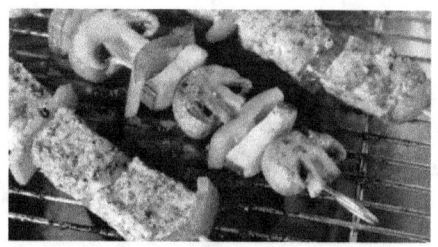

The fizz on alcohol – If you do happen to crave or want to delight in an occasional alcoholic beverage, stick to clear spirits such as vodka, tequila or gin. They are low in carbs and can be mixed with soda rather than fruit juices. A martini is actually encouraged within the rulebook of the Atkins diet. If you fancy a glass of wine, opt for the white over the red.

Truly understand what you are eating – The basic principle of the Atkins diet is learning to eat right. That is one of the main reasons that the Atkins diet is implemented in four phases. Through each phase, you grasp more and more knowledge about what you are fueling your body with. You understand which foods help you lose or gain weight and how to reduce the consuming of empty calories.

Be sensible in regards to portions – There is no need to count the calories you intake while on Atkins, but you still need to keep your common sense intact. It is no secret that too many calories will slow down your weight loss progress. But did you know that consuming too few calories can actually hurt you metabolism, which is the main conductor on the train to losing weight?

Learn how to enjoy eating anywhere – Unlike many other diets that put such restrictions on what participants consume, on the Atkins Diet, you are allowed to eat out or at a friends' house. Atkins encourages the consumption of whole foods, especially delicious ones! You will learn how to pick the right types of foods that feed your body the correct way, in ways that calories burn faster than fire. This means dining and out or eating at other locations other than just at home will be challenging at first, but you will become seasoned in the ways of picking foods that fuel you in the healthiest ways.

Learn how to plan ahead – Learn how to properly stock your kitchen cupboards and pantry with the right foods that keep you motivated. Get rid of items that you know will throw you off your dieting course. Also, it is a good idea to become accustomed to planning out meals, so that when you step into the grocery store to start shopping you can have a one-track mind and don't get veered away by other things you should not be consuming.

Take supplements – Along with the consumption of whole-rich foods, supplements may be necessary to ensure that your body is receiving the proper amount of nutrients it needs to function at its most prime. Taking a daily multivitamin is your best bet, one with potassium, magnesium and calcium, but skip the iron, unless you already have a deficiency, of course. Consuming fish oil is a good alternative to receive a good amount of healthy omega-3s too.

Cheating is okay – Many other diets leave participants in a panic when they have gone and cheated, making them feel guilty, which only fuels bad eating habits more. Whether in the Atkins or another diet, the world will not coming to a screeching halt if you accidentally consume something you aren't supposed to. If you cheat, you are fine! It may set you back a day or two, but the Atkins diet makes it so darn easy to get back upon the weight loss train! We are human, we are expected to mess up a time or two, or cheat on our diets.

Encourage support – Let you family and friends know of your new mission and lifestyle changes, and you will be surprised the support you will receive in return! If you hide your dieting changes, it is only going to become harder to stick to them, and can easily lead you to a path that ends in failure. There are also online forums and in-person Atkins groups that meet in specific areas if you need an extra boost to keep yourself on track! Meeting and communicating with other people who are also taking the Atkins challenge can be a great motivator. The Atkins Community Forum can be found at community.atkins.com/index.jsp

Chapter 5: Breakfast Recipes

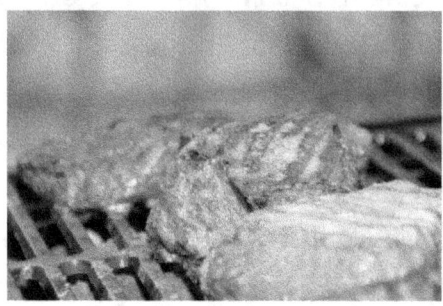

Breakfast is the most important meal of the day, and on the Atkins diet it is no different! Eating a good breakfast jump starts our bodies for the day, leading us to make a better decision in what we eat. This chapter is filled with a few delicious recipes to get your day started the Atkins way!

One Minute Coconut And Almond Muffins

Prep: 3 minutes
Cook Time: 1 minute
Phase: 2

9.7 grams protein
3 grams fiber
16.8 grams fat
207 calories

What's in it:

1 tsp. extra virgin olive oil
1 egg
1/8 tsp. salt
¼ tsp. baking powder
½ tsp. cinnamon
1 tsp. Sucralose based sweetener
1/3 tsp. organic high fiber coconut flour
2 tbsp. almond meal flour

How it's made:

- In a coffee mug, pour in all the dry ingredients, combine thoroughly.
- Add the oil and egg, stirring until well combined.
- Put mug in microwave and heat for 1 minute. Using a knife, remove the muffin from cup, slice and butter to your heart's content
- Enjoy!

Pineapple-Almond Smoothie

Prep: 5 minutes
Phase: 3

10.8 grams protein

4.2 grams fiber
18.6 grams fat
280 calories

What's in it:

½ c. Pure Almond Milk – Unsweetened
20 whole slivered and blanched almonds
2 ½ ounces of pineapple
½ c. of plain yogurt

How it's made:

- Combine almond milk, almonds, pineapple and yogurt in a blender, proceeding to puree until mixture is creamy and smooth in texture.
  o (You may use other fruits and nuts. Ensure that you use fresh pineapple to ensure a great tasting smoothie!)

Almond And Blueberry Pancakes

Prep: 5 minutes
Cook time: 10 minutes
Phase: 2

20.3 grams protein
2.5 grams fiber
10 grams fat

212 calories

What's in it:

¼ c. blueberries
2 tbsp. vanilla whey protein
½ ounce of creamed cottage cheese
¼ tsp. baking powder
1/8 c. dry whole grain soy flour
¾ large egg
1/16 c. almond flour, blanched

How it's made:

- Mix together baking powder, soy flour, protein powder and almond flour. Then proceed to mix in the beaten egg and cottage cheese until thoroughly combined.
- Lightly grease a nonstick skillet over medium heat
- Utilizing about ¼ c. per pancake made, drop batter on skillet. When you see bubbles start to appear in middle, turn over and cook an additional 2 minutes until firm
- Serve along with blueberries

Jack Cheese, Avocado And Bacon Omelets With Freshly Made Salsa

Prep: 10 minutes
Cook time: 10 minutes
Phase: 1

33 grams protein
3.9 grams fiber
42.5 grams fat
553 calories

What's in it:

1 c. Monterey jack cheese, shredded
½ avocado
1 tbsp. unsalted butter
3 medium slices of bacon, cooked
1 ounce of water
4 eggs
1 tbsp. fresh lime juice
1 ounce of cilantro
½ c. jalapeño peppers
3 medium scallions
1 medium red tomato

How it's made:

- To prepare salsa, dice up tomatoes, green onion and jalapeño. Combine tomato, green onions, jalapeño, cilantro and lime juice in a small bowl, stirring well to thoroughly combine. Season with salt and pepper to taste, then set aside
- Whisk together eggs and water in a bowl, seasoning with salt and pepper. Prepare bacon, crumble and set to the side
- In a skillet over medium-high heat, melt half the butter, adding in egg mixture when foaming subsides. Sprinkle half the mixture with bacon, avocado and cheese, and proceed to cook for a minute
- Fold over in skillet, then plate omelet. Serve with freshly made salsa and enjoy!

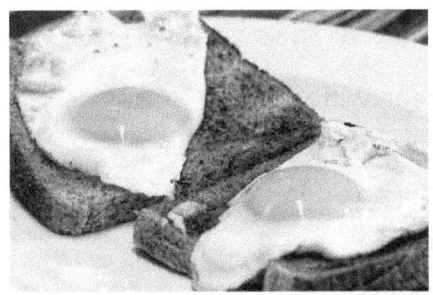

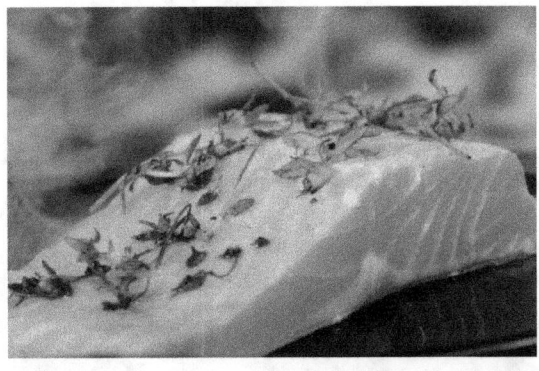

Chapter 6: Lunch Recipes

Macho Chili

Prep: 10 minutes
Cook time: 165 minutes
Phase: 1

43.9 grams protein
1.4 grams fiber
12.4 grams fat
325 calories

What's in it:

6 ounces red wine
14 ½ ounces of red tomatoes
3 tbsp. chili powder
2 tsp. garlic
1 medium onion
3 tbsp. extra virgin olive oil
½ tsp black pepper
2 tsp. salt
5 pounds of beef top sirloin

How it's made:

- Ensure that your oven is preheated to 325 degrees
- Season beef with both salt and pepper
- In a Dutch oven, heat oil over high heat, proceeding to add 1/3 of beef, browning all sides, which takes around 60 seconds per side
- Transfer cooked meat to bowl and repeat until all sides of meat is cooked
- Chop up the onion and add into the Dutch oven with remaining oil. Cook garlic and onion until lightly browned. Pour in wine, tomatoes and chili powder, bringing to a simmer.
- Return beef to Dutch oven, cover and back for 2.5 hours, ensuring that you stir halfway through your cook time, until beat is tender.
- One serving equals about ¾-1 cup

Chapter 7: Dinner Recipes

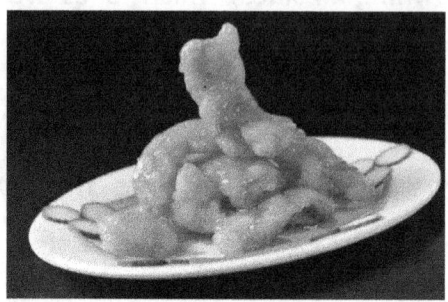

These dinner recipes are for sure going to satisfy your stomach and taste buds alike, without that gut wrenching feeling of being too full!

Apricot Glazed Brisket

Prep: 10 minutes
Cook time: 210 minutes
Phase: 2

47.1 grams protein
0.3 grams fiber
16.8 grams fat
358 calories

What's in it:

3 tbsp. Sugar-free apricot preserves

1 tsp. black pepper

2 tsp. paprika

1 tsp. salt

4 pounds beef brisket (whole, lean only)

How it's made:

- Ensure your oven is preheated to 475 degrees. Season brisket with pepper, salt and paprika
- In a Dutch over, place your brisket fat side down, placing onions and carrots around meat. Cook for 15 minutes
- Proceed to turn your brisket fat side up and add about ½ cup of water. Tightly cover Dutch oven. Ensure that you reduce over temperature to 375 degrees.
- Cook for 3-4 hours, until the brisket is tender with the touch of a fork
- Turn on the broiler. Remove brisket from the depths of the Dutch over and place into a broiler pan.
- Spread apricot preserves over brisket, proceeding to broil for 5 minutes, until jam is lightly brown in color in most areas. Remove carrots and onions from cooking juices while meat is in broiler
- Cover brisket with follow and allow at least 15 minutes for meat to rest before attempting to serve. Serve with cooking juices. Enjoy!

Bacon Wrapped Filet With Blue Cheese Butter Sauce

Prep: 15 minutes
Cook time: 45 minutes
Phase: 1

54.5 grams protein
4 grams fiber
36.2 grams fat
581 calories

What's in it:

¼ tsp black pepper
¼ tsp. salt
2 tsp. olive oil
8 ounces of baby spinach
1/3 tbsp. red wine vinegar
3 ounce of blue cheese
1 tbsp. unsalted butter
2 slices bacon
12 oz beef tenderloin
3 cherry tomatoes
4 ounce Portobello mushroom cap
2 medium green onions

How it's made:

- Ensure that your oven is preheated to 425 degrees.
- Finely chop the green portion of the onions and throw in a small bowl. Dice the white part of the onion and set aside. Remove cap from mushroom, throwing away the stem portion. Chop the mushroom cap into ¼" pieces, set aside
- Pat the beef dry with a paper towel. Slice meat half widthwise and press on each half to make into filet mignon steaks. Season the filets with salt and pepper. Proceed to wrap edges with bacon slices. Set aside
- Add butter and an ounce of blue cheese in with the green portion of chopped onions and combine well.
- In a separate bowl, mix together red wine vinegar, salt and pepper, slowing whisking in olive oil, set aside
- In a nonstick skillet over medium-high heat, heat up 2 teaspoons of olive oil, adding in steaks when hot. Ensure that you sear all sides of steaks, frequently turning with tongs until brown, 3 minutes per side.
- Put on a sheet lined in foil and roast for 6-8 minutes
- While meat is roasting, add mushrooms and white part of onion with salt and pepper in a sauté pan on low heat. Sauté until mushrooms are tender.
- Put spinach in a bowl and add rest of blue cheese, drizzling vinaigrette over the spinach leaves, toss to combine
- Spoon mushrooms on two plates, topping with cooked fillet and blue cheese butter. Enjoy!

Chapter 8: Dessert Recipes

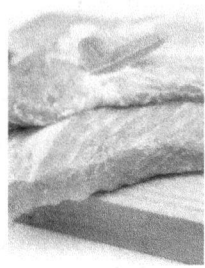

With these delectable dessert recipes, you will forget you are on any kind of a diet as your taste buds scream for joy!

Raspberry-Almond Cupcakes

Prep: 15 minutes
Cook time: 25 minutes
Phase: 2

7.4 grams protein
4 grams fiber
20.7 grams fat
236 calories

What's in it:

3 1/3 tbsp. Sugar-free red raspberry preserves
½ tsp. salt

½ tsp. baking powder

2 ½ c. almond meal flour

2 tsp. pure almond extract

1 tsp. vanilla extract

½ tsp. fresh lemon juice

1 ounce water

2 tbsp heavy cream

1/3 c. sucralose based sweetener

¼ c. unsalted butter

2 large eggs

How it's made:

- Ensure that your oven is preheated to 350 degrees. In a muffin tin, place paper cupcake liners and set aside.
- Beat egg yolks and ¼ cup of sucralose, water, cream, lemon juice and both extracts in a small bowl together until thoroughly combined. Set aside.
- Beat egg whites until they are frothy in a separate bowl, then add the remaining sucralose, beating until nice and stiff peaks take shape. Fold egg whites gently into the egg yolk mixture.
- Mix together salt, baking powder and almond meal in another bowl. Proceed to fold gently into the egg mixture.
- Divide batter equally among muffin cups
- Drop 1 tsp. of raspberry preserves into the center of each
- Bake cupcakes for 20-30 minutes, until a toothpick comes out clean when inserted into the center.

- Allow cupcakes to cook for at least 20 minutes, you can enjoy warm or at room temperature. Chill remaining cupcakes for up to a week, or freeze for up to one month.

Atkins Brownies

Prep: 15 minutes
Cook time: 30 minutes
Phase: 2

6.6 grams protein
1.2 grams fiber
9.4 grams fat
119 calories

What's in it:

4 ½ serving of all purpose low-carb baking mix
2 tbsp. baking powder
1 c. sucralose based sweetener
5 large eggs
½ c. heavy cream
½ c. unsalted butter
4 ounces of unsweetened baking chocolate squares

How it's made:

- Ensure that your oven is preheated to 325 degrees.

- In a bowl, microwave unsweetened chocolate and butter together for 2 minutes until melted, proceed to whisk in the heavy cream.
- Add eggs and 1 cup of sugar substitute into a bowl. Beat with electric mixer until blended
- Reducing mixing speed to low, add in chocolate mixture
- Mix in baking powder and low carb baking mix
- Grease an 8x8 baking pan, and proceed to pour batter evenly inside
- Bake brownies for 30-35 minutes until done
- Let brownies cool, cut and enjoy!

Chocolate Ginger Cake

Prep: 20 minutes
Cook time: 45 minutes
Phase: 2

6.6 grams protein
2.2 grams fiber
15.6 grams fat
185 calories

What's in it:

¼ tsp. cream of tartar
2 tsp. ground ginger
12 large eggs

2 ¼ c. sucralose
¼ c. whole grain soy flour
¼ c. unsweetened cocoa powder
1/3 c. canola oil
1/3 cup water
4 ounces of unsweetened baking chocolate squares
¾ c. pecan halves

How it's made:

- Ensure that your oven is preheated to 350 degrees.
- Toast pecans for 8 minutes on a cookie sheet, proceeding to coarsely chop them up. Then set aside.
- Ensure that you lower over to 325 degrees. Grease the bottom of a 10 inch in tubular pan, lining with parchment paper
- In a microwavable bowl, heat chocolate and water for 1-2 minutes until melted, checking in intervals of 30 seconds-1 minute. Stir until smooth. Cool until chocolate is lukewarm, then stir in oil, set aside.
- Pulse soy flour, cocoa powder and pecans in a food processor until finely ground.
- Beat egg yolks and sugar substitute in a large bowl with an electric mixer on high speed, until mixture is light and fluffy in texture, which takes about 5 minutes. Proceed to stir in melted chocolate, ginger and your pecan mixture.
- Beat egg whites and cream of tartar in another large bowl on medium speed with mixer, until frothy looking. Proceed to gradually add sugar, beating until stiff peaks appear.

- Fold in a third of the meringue into the yolk mixture to lighten, and then proceed to fold in the remainder of the meringue until thoroughly combined
- Pour batter in prepared pan evenly.
- Bake for 45 minutes, until a toothpick inserted in middle of cake comes out clean
- Allow the cake 30 minutes to cool before attempting to remove from the pan
- Run a knife around the outer and inner rims of cake and place on wire rack.
- Allow to cool completely before serving.

Chapter 9: Entree Recipes

Almond-Raspberry Cupcakes

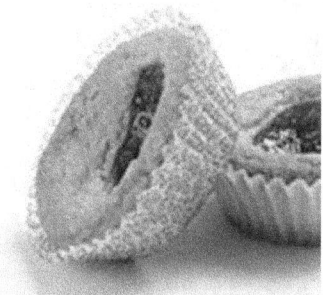

Servings: 10 | **Prep:** 15 m | **Style:** American | **Cook:** 25 m

Ingredients
- 2 large Eggs (Whole)
- 1/4 cup Unsalted Butter Stick
- 1/3 cup Sucralose Based Sweetener (Sugar Substitute)
- 2 tbsps Heavy Cream
- 1 fl oz Tap Water
- 1/2 tsp Fresh Lemon Juice
- 1 tsp Vanilla Extract
- 2 tsps Pure Almond Extract
- 2 1/2 cups Almond Meal Flour
- 1/2 tsp Baking Powder (Straight Phosphate, Double Acting)
- 1/2 tsp Salt
- 3 1/3 tbsps Sugar Free Red Raspberry Preserves

Directions

1. Preheat oven to 350°F. Place 10 paper cups in a muffin pan and set aside. In a small bowl beat the egg yolks with 1/4 cup sucralose, butter, cream, water, lemon juice or vinegar and extracts until fully combined. Set aside.
2. In another bowl beat the egg whites until frothy, add the remaining 2 tablespoons of sucralose and continue to beat until stiff peaks form. Gently fold the egg whites into the egg yolk mixture.
3. In a separate bowl, combine the almond meal, baking powder and salt. Gently fold into the egg mixture. Divide this batter equally between the muffin cups then drop 1 teaspoon of raspberry jam into the center.
4. Bake for 20-30 minutes until a toothpick inserted in the center comes out clean. Allow to cool in the pan for 20 minutes. Enjoy warm or at room temperature. Refrigerate remaining cupcakes in an airtight container for up t0 one week and serve at room temperature. These may also be frozen for up to 1 month.

Nutritional Information
- Protein : 7.4g
- Fat : 20.7g
- Fiber : 4g
- Calories :236

Apricot-Glazed Brisket

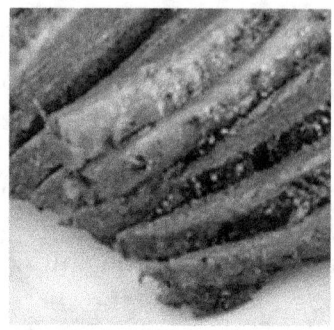

Servings: 8 | **Prep:** 10 m | **Style:** American | **Cook:** 210 m

Ingredients
- 4 lbs Beef Brisket (Whole, Lean Only)
- 2 tsps Salt
- 2 tsps Paprika
- 1 tsp Black Pepper
- 3 tbsps Sugar Free Apricot Preserves

Directions
1. Heat oven to 475F. Season brisket with salt, paprika and pepper.
2. Place brisket fat side down in a Dutch oven. Scatter onions and carrots around the beef. Cook 15 minutes.
3. Turn brisket fat side up and add 1/2 cup water. Cover tightly. Reduce oven temperature to 375°F. Cook 3 to 4 hours, until brisket is fork tender.
4. Heat broiler. Remove brisket from Dutch oven and place on a broiler pan. Spread jam over brisket. Broil 6 from heat source

5 minutes, until jam is lightly browned in spots. While brisket is broiling, remove onions and carrots from cooking juices.
5. Cover brisket with foil and allow to rest 15 minutes before serving. Remove surface fat with a spoon and serve with degreased cooking juices.

Nutritional Information
- Protein : 47.1g
- Fat : 16.8g
- Fiber : 0.3g
- Calories :358

Artichokes With Lemon-Butter

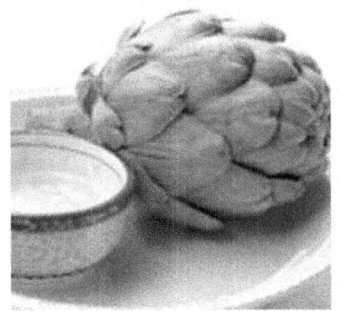

Servings: 4 | **Prep:** 10 m | **Style:** American | **Cook:** 15 m

Ingredients
- 4 medium Artichokes (Globe or French)
- 4 fruit (2-1/8" dia) Lemon
- 2 tbsps Coriander Seed
- 2 tbsps Salt

- 1/2 cup Unsalted Butter Stick

Directions
1. Bring 4 quarts of water to a boil in a large pot. Trim the stems of the artichokes to about 2 inches.
2. Halve 3 lemons and squeeze juice into water. Add lemon halves, coriander seeds and salt. Place artichokes in the cooking liquid, and cover with a heavy plate to keep them from floating. Boil 15 minutes, until a paring knife, inserted where the stem meets the bottom, comes out easily. Remove and drain excess water.
3. In a small bowl, melt butter in a microwave or saucepan. Mix in juice of remaining lemon, salt and pepper.
4. Serve each person one whole artichoke, accompanied by a ramekin of butter sauce and a large bowl for discarded leaves. Season with freshly ground salt and pepper to taste.

Nutritional Information
- Protein : 4.8g
- Fat : 23.7g
- Fiber : 10g
- Calories :287

Arugula, Pear And Hazelnut Salad

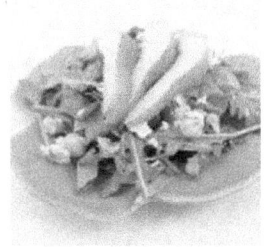

Servings: 4 | **Prep**: 10 m | **Style**: American

Ingredients
- 10 oz Arugula (Rocket)
- 1/2 cup crumbled Gorgonzola Cheese
- 2 servings Maple-Dijon Vinaigrette
- 1 medium (approx 2-1/2 per lb) Pears
- 40 nuts Hazelnuts or Filberts

Directions
1. Use the Atkins recipe to make Maple-Dijon Vinaigrette for this recipe. You will need 4 Tbsp. This salad is delicious served with salmon.
2. Toast hazelnuts in a dry skillet for about 15 minutes or toast on a sheet pan in an oven at 350°F (stir 2-3 times for both methods); allow to cool and gently rub off outer skin, coarsely chop, and set aside.
3. Make the Maple-Dijon Vinaigrette and toss 4 tablespoons with the arugula and Gorgonzola cheese. Transfer to serving plates.
4. Arrange the pear slices in a fan on top and sprinkle with hazelnuts.

Nutritional Information
- Protein : 7.1g
- Fat : 20g
- Fiber : 4.4g
- Calories :244

Asian Beef Salad With Edamame

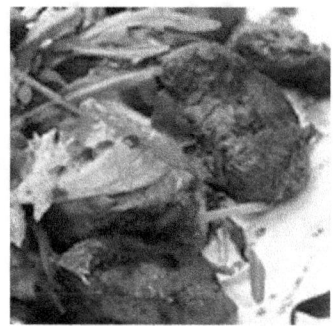

Servings: 1 | **Prep:** 720 m | **Style:** Asian | **Cook:** 5 m

Ingredients
- medium (4-1/8" long) Scallions or Spring Onions
- 1/4 tsp Garlic
- 1/2 tbsp Tamari Soybean Sauce
- 1/4 tbsp Sodium and Sugar Free Rice Vinegar
- 1/4 tsp Toasted Sesame Oil
- 1/8 tsp Sucralose Based Sweetener (Sugar Substitute)
- 4 1/4 oz Beef Top Sirloin (Trimmed to 1/8" Fat, Choice Grade)

- 1/8 tsp Curry Powder
- 1/16 tsp Ginger (Ground)
- 1/2 tbsp Canola Vegetable Oil
- 3/4 cup Spring Mix Salad
- 1/4 medium (approx 2-3/4" long, 2-1/2" dia) Red Sweet Pepper
- 2 oz Waterchestnuts
- 1/2 cup Shelled Edamame

Directions

Note: Because only half of the marinade is used in this recipe for the salad dressing and the rest is used as a marinade and discarded, please double the first six ingredients. (The nutritionals shown are correct.) For added flavor, use dark (toasted) sesame oil instead of regular sesame oil.

1. Mix green onions, garlic, soy sauce, rice wine vinegar, sesame oil and sugar substitute in a small bowl. Pour half into a resealable plastic bag; add steak and marinate overnight in the refrigerator.
2. To remaining soy sauce mixture, add curry powder and ground ginger. Heat canola oil in a large skillet over high heat until very hot.
3. Drain beef and discard marinade; quickly stir-fry beef 2 to 3 minutes in hot oil. Transfer to a large mixing bowl. Add salad greens, bell pepper, water chestnuts, edamame and reserved soy dressing. Toss to coat.

Nutritional Information
- Protein : 37.5g

- Fat : 16.3g
- Fiber : 8.1g
- Calories :395

Asian Beef Salad With Sesame Seeds

Servings: 1 | **Prep:** 720 m | **Style:** Asian | **Cook:** 5 m

Ingredients
- 1/4 tsp Garlic
- 1/2 tbsp Tamari Soybean Sauce
- 1/8 tbsp Sodium and Sugar Free Rice Vinegar
- 1/4 tsp Sesame Oil
- 1/8 tsp Sucralose Based Sweetener (Sugar Substitute)
- 1/8 tsp Curry Powder
- 1/16 tsp Ginger (Ground)
- 4 1/4 oz Beef Top Sirloin (Trimmed to 1/8" Fat, Choice Grade)
- 1 cup Spring Mix Salad
- 1/2 tbsp Canola Vegetable Oil
- 1/4 large (2-1/4 per lb, approx 3-3/4" long, 3" dia) Sweet Red Peppers
- 2 oz Waterchestnuts
- 1 tbsp Dried Whole Sesame Seeds
- 1 large Scallions or Spring Onion

Directions

Note: Because only half of the marinade is used in this recipe for the salad dressing and the rest is used as a marinade and discarded, please double the first six ingredients. (The nutritionals shown are correct.) For added flavor, use dark (toasted) sesame oil instead of regular sesame oil.

1. Mix green onions, garlic, soy sauce, rice wine vinegar, sesame oil and granular sugar substitute in a small bowl. Pour half into a resealable plastic bag; add steak and marinate overnight in the refrigerator.
2. To remaining soy sauce mixture, add curry powder and ginger. Heat canola oil in a large skillet over high heat until very hot.
3. Drain beef and discard marinade; quickly stir-fry beef 2 to 3 minutes in hot oil for medium doneness. Transfer to a large mixing bowl. Add salad greens, bell pepper, water chestnuts and reserved soy dressing. Toss to coat. Sprinkle with sesame seeds.

Nutritional Information
- Protein : 31.9g
- Fat : 20.1g
- Fiber : 6.1g
- Calories :375

Asian Lobster Salad

Servings: 2 | **Prep:** 15 m | **Style:** Asian

Ingredients
- 3/4 lb Northern Lobster
- 2 cups shredded Chinese Cabbage (Bok-Choy, Pak-Choi)
- 1/2 small Sweet Red Pepper

- 4 medium (4-1/8" long) Scallions or Spring Onions
- 1 tbsp Dried Whole Sesame Seeds
- 2 tbsps Sodium and Sugar Free Rice Vinegar
- 2 tbsps Tamari Soybean Sauce
- 1 tbsp Canola Vegetable Oil
- 1 tsp Sesame Oil
- 1 tsp Ginger

Directions
1. For the salad: In a large serving bowl, combine lobster, cabbage, bell pepper, scallions and sesame seeds.
2. For the dressing: In a small bowl, whisk the rice vinegar, Tamari soy sauce, ginger and sesame and canola oils together.
3. Pour dressing over salad and toss gently to coat. Season with fresh ground black pepper and salt.

Nutritional Information
- Protein : 39.8g
- Fat : 14g
- Fiber : 3g
- Calories :325

Asian Marinade

Servings: 6 | **Prep:** 5 m | **Style:** Asian

Ingredients
- 8 tbsps Tamari Soybean Sauce
- 2 tbsps Sodium and Sugar Free Rice Vinegar
- 2 tbsps Xylitol
- 1 tbsp Ginger

- 1 tsp Garlic
- 2 tsps Toasted Sesame Oil
- 2 tbsps Canola Vegetable Oil

Directions

Try this simple marinade with chicken kebabs, salmon or tuna steaks, pork chops or beef tenderloin. Marinate chicken and meat for up to 24 hours in the refrigerator, fish for up to 2 hours. Each serving is 2 Tbsp.

1. Combine tamari, vinegar, sugar substitute, ginger, garlic and sesame oil in a bowl. Slowly whisk in canola oil until combined.

Nutritional Information
- Protein : 2.6g
- Fat : 6,3g
- Fiber : 4.2g
- Calories :81

Asian Steak Salad

Servings: 2 | **Style:** Asian | **Cook:** 45 m

Ingredients
- clove Garlic
- 2 large Young Green Onions
- 1/4 oz Ginger

- 1 medium (approx 2-3/4" long, 2-1/2" dia) Red Sweet Pepper
- 1 tbsp Organic Tamari
- 1/2 tbsp Unseasoned Rice Wine Vinegar
- 1/2 tsp Sesame Oil
- 1/4 tsp No Calorie Sweetener
- 8 oz Beef Top Sirloin (Trimmed to 1/8" Fat)
- 1/4 tsp Curry Powder
- 1 tbsp Vegetable Oil
- 5 oz Baby Spinach

Directions
1. Finely chop the garlic and place in a medium bowl. Finely chop the green onions and add to the garlic. Peel and grate the ginger and place in a small bowl. Remove the stem, pith and seeds from the red bell pepper and discard. Cut into ¼-inch thin strips; set aside.
2. To the medium bowl with the garlic and green onions, add tamari sauce, rice wine vinegar, sesame oil and sugar substitute and stir until well combined. Pour HALF of the tamari mixture into the ziplock bag; set aside.
3. Pat dry the sirloin steak with paper towels and cut into ⅛-inch slices. Place in the bag with the marinade. Seal the bag tightly and place in the refrigerator to marinate. To the tamari mixture remaining in the medium bowl add the curry powder and the ginger; hold for step 5.
4. Heat 1 tablespoon of canola oil in a large sauté pan over medium-high heat. When the pan is hot, remove the steak from the marinade, and quickly stir-fry for 2 to 3 minutes until the beef is cooked through (Discard the marinade). Transfer the steak to a large bowl,
5. Add the red pepper, baby spinach the reserved tamari mixture. Toss to coat all ingredients well.
6. Divide the Asian Beef Salad between two plates and enjoy!

Nutritional Information
- Protein : 27.3g
- Fat : 22.9g
- Fiber : 3.5g
- Calories :351

Asian Tuna Kebabs

Servings: 8 | **Prep:** 25 m | **Style:** Asian | **Cook:** 8 m

Ingredients
- 5 1/3 tbsps Tamari Gluten Free Soy Sauce
- 2 2/3 fl ozs Rice Wine
- 1 tbsp Toasted Sesame Oil
- 1 tbsp Ginger
- 3 tsps Garlic
- 2 tsps Sucralose Based Sweetener (Sugar Substitute)
- 32 oz boneless Tuna
- 3 large Scallions or Spring Onions
- 1 large (2.25 per pound, approx 3-3/4" long, 3" dia) Red Sweet Pepper
- 3/4 lb Eggplant

Directions

You'll need 8 bamboo skewers, which should be soaked in water for 15 minutes before cooking. Or use metal skewers. Chinese eggplants are thinner and less bitter than Italian ones and can be found in Asian markets or well-stocked produce sections of most supermarkets.

1. Heat grill to high.
2. Combine soy sauce, rice wine, sesame oil, ginger, garlic and sugar substitute in a large bowl.
3. Add tuna, scallions and red pepper and toss to coat. Marinate for 15 minutes in the refrigerator. Remove tuna, scallions and red pepper from marinade and set aside.
4. Toss eggplant in marinade and let sit for 3 minutes. Remove eggplant and set aside with other ingredients. Discard marinade.
5. Thread skewers, alternating 3 pieces of tuna, 2 pieces of scallions, 2 pieces of red pepper and 3 pieces of eggplant on each. Eggplant should be skewered through both skin sides of the rounds.
6. Grill for 3 -4 minutes per side tuna will be rare in the center.

Nutritional Information
- Protein : 28.7g
- Fat : 7.5g
- Fiber : 2.2g
- Calories :221

Asian Vegetable Bowl

Servings: 6 | **Prep**: 10 m | **Style**: Asian | **Cook:** 10 m

Ingredients
- 3 cups chopped Scallions or Spring Onions
- 2 cups Mushroom Pieces and Stems
- 4 tbsps Tamari Soybean Sauce
- 3 tsps Ginger

- 1 clove Garlic
- 1 pepper Serrano Pepper
- 1 cup chopped or sliced Red Tomato
- 6 oz Firm Silken Tofu
- 1 carrot (7-1/2") Carrots
- 1/2 oz Cilantro (Coriander)
- 2 cups shredded Chinese Cabbage (Bok-Choy, Pak-Choi)
- 6 cups Chicken Broth, Bouillon or Consomme

Directions
1. To make this soup suitable for earlier phases, simply omit the carrot. Also vegetable broth may be substituted for the chicken broth to make it appropriate for Vegetarians and Vegans.
2. In a large saucepan, bring broth and tamari to a boil.
3. Reduce heat; add bok choy, mushrooms, ginger, garlic (minced) and chili. Simmer for 5 minutes, until bok choy is tender but still crisp and mushrooms are softened.
4. Add tomatoes, green onions, tofu and carrot. Heat through for 1 minute.
5. Stir in cilantro just before serving.

Nutritional Information
- Protein : 6.7g
- Fat : 2.1g
- Fiber : 1.8g
- Calories :65

Asian Veggie And Pork Bowl

Servings: 2 | **Prep:** 10 m | **Style:** Asian | **Cook:** 45 m

Ingredients
- 4 medium (4-1/8" long) Young Green Onions
- 1/4 oz Cilantro (Coriander)
- 4 oz Brown Mushrooms (Crimini Italian)
- 1/4 oz Ginger
- 1 clove Garlic
- 1/2 pepper Serrano Pepper
- 5 oz Chinese Cabbage (Bok-Choy, Pak-Choi)
- 1 italian Tomato
- 8 oz Pork Loin (Tenderloin)
- 1 cube Chicken Stock Cubes (Dry, Dehydrated)
- 1 tbsp Organic Tamari
- 1 tbsp Vegetable Oil

Directions
1. Slice the green onions into ¼-inch pieces on a bias; set aside. Remove the stems from the crimini mushrooms and discard stems. Cut the mushrooms into ¼-inch slices; set aside. Remove the cilantro leaves from the stems and discard stems. Roughly chop the cilantro and set aside.
2. Peel the ginger and finely chop; set aside. Finely chop the garlic cloves; set aside. Remove the stem, pith and seeds from only HALF of the Serrano chile and discard. Finely chop and set aside. Remove the end of the baby bok choy and cut into very thin slices lengthwise; set aside. Cut the tomato in half lengthwise. Cut each half into three wedges; set aside.
3. Pat dry the pork tenderloin with paper towels. Cut into ¼-inch thin slices. Heat a medium sauté pan with 1 tablespoon of canola oil over medium-high heat. When hot, add the pork tenderloin slices and sear for 2 to 3 minutes until browned and cooked through. Remove the pork from the pan and set aside.
4. Bring the chicken stock concentrate, tamari sauce and 2 cups of water to a boil in a large sauce pot over high heat. Reduce

the heat to medium-high, add the mushrooms, ginger, garlic, serrano and the baby bok choy. Simmer for 5 minutes, until the bok choy is tender but still crisp and the mushrooms are softened.
5. Add the tomatoes, green onions and the pork to the sauce pot. Heat through for 1 minute. Remove from heat and stir in the cilantro.
6. Ladle the soup into two bowls. Enjoy!

Nutritional Information
- Protein : 28.2g
- Fat : 13.4g
- Fiber : 2.6g
- Calories :270

Asian-Style Coleslaw

Servings: 6 | **Prep**: 15 m | **Style:** Asian

Ingredients
- 1 large (7-1/4" to 8-1/2" long) Carrots
- 1 cup chopped Snowpeas (Pea Pod)
- 12 oz Chinese Cabbage (Bok-Choy, Pak-Choi)
- 2 tbsps Extra Virgin Olive Oil
- 1 tbsp Toasted Sesame Oil
- 2 tbsps Sodium and Sugar Free Rice Vinegar
- 1 tbsp Tamari Soybean Sauce
- 2 tsps Ginger
- 1 tsp Sucralose Based Sweetener (Sugar Substitute)

Directions

1. To make this suitable for earlier phases, simply eliminate the carrot.
2. Place cabbage in a large bowl; grate carrot into cabbage. Mix in snow peas.
3. In a small bowl, mix oils, vinegar, tamari, ginger and sugar substitute.
4. Pour dressing over salad; toss to coat. Season to taste with salt.

Nutritional Information
- Protein : 1.7g
- Fat : 7g
- Fiber : 1.4g
- Calories :82

Asparagus And Leek Soup

Servings: 4 | **Prep:** 15 m | **Style:** Other | **Cook:** 15 m

Ingredients
- 2 tbsps Unsalted Butter Stick
- 1 leek Leeks
- 3/4 lb Asparagus
- 1 tsp Garlic
- 1 14.5 oz can Chicken Broth, Bouillon or Consomme
- 1/3 cup Heavy Cream

Directions
1. Melt butter in a large pot over medium-high heat. Add leeks and sauté for 3 minutes. Add asparagus and cook 1 minute more. Add garlic and sauté for 30 more seconds.
2. Add broth to pot and bring to a boil.

3. Lower heat, cover and simmer 8 to 10 minutes, until asparagus is tender.
4. Mix in cream, salt and pepper. Blend soup in a food processor or blender until smooth.
5. Return to pot to heat through before serving (if necessary). Season with salt and freshly ground black pepper to taste.

Nutritional Information
- Protein : 3.3g
- Fat : 13.5g
- Fiber : 2.2g
- Calories :156

Asparagus In Vinaigrette With Walnuts

Servings: 4 | **Prep:** 10 m | **Style:** American | **Cook:** 10 m

Ingredients
- 1 lb Asparagus
- 1/4 small Onion
- 2 tbsps White Wine Vinegar
- 1 tsp Dijon Mustard
- 1/2 individual packet Sucralose Based Sweetener (Sugar Substitute)
- 1/2 tsp Salt
- 1/4 tsp Black Pepper
- 1/4 cup Extra Virgin Olive Oil
- 4 cups Spring Mix Salad
- 1/4 cup chopped English Walnuts

Directions

1. To toast nuts, place them on a baking sheet in a preheated 325°F oven, turning them after 3 minutes. Bake for another 3 to 6 minutes, checking frequently to avoid burning. You can substitute almonds for walnuts, if you prefer. To make this dish suitable for Induction, simply eliminate the walnuts.
2. Steam asparagus until crisp-tender, about 4-7 minutes, depending upon size. Drain, and pat dry with paper towels. Set aside.
3. Combine white onion, vinegar, mustard, sugar substitute, salt and pepper in a mixing bowl. Gradually whisk in oil.
4. Divide lettuce on 4 plates; arrange asparagus on top and drizzle with vinaigrette. Sprinkle with walnuts and additional salt and pepper, if desired.

Nutritional Information
- Protein : 4.3g
- Fat : 18.8g
- Fiber : 4.4g
- Calories :206

Asparagus Tarragon Cream Soup

Servings: 8 | **Prep:** 25 m | **Style:** Other | **Cook:** 30 m

Ingredients
- 1 tbsp Extra Virgin Olive Oil
- 3 14.5 oz cans Chicken Broth, Bouillon or Consomme
- 2 lbs Asparagus
- 3 stalk medium (7-1/2" - 8" long) Celery
- 1/4 tsp Salt
- 1/4 tsp Black Pepper
- 1 small Onion
- 1/2 tbsp leaf Tarragon

- 3/4 cup Heavy Cream

Directions
1. Heat oil in a large pot over medium-high heat. Add white onion and cook 5 minutes, until softened but not browned.
2. Add broth, asparagus, celery, salt, pepper and half of the tarragon to the pot. Bring to a boil.
3. Lower heat, cover and simmer 20 minutes, until asparagus is very tender.
4. In a blender, puré soup in batches until smooth. Return to pot. Add cream and remaining tarragon and heat soup through over medium heat. Season with salt and freshly ground black pepper.

Nutritional Information
- Protein : 3.9g
- Fat : 10.5g
- Fiber : 2.9g
- Calories :128

Asparagus Wrapped In Chili Spiced Bacon

Servings: 4 | **Prep:** 20 m | **Style:** American | **Cook:** 12 m

Ingredients
- 1 tsp Chili Powder
- 1/2 tsp Sucralose Based Sweetener (Sugar Substitute)
- 4 slices Bacon
- 24 spears Asparagus

Directions

1. Soak 16 wooden toothpicks in warm water for 20 minutes.
2. Preheat grill. Place a sheet of wax paper on a sheet pan and set aside. Combine the chili powder and sugar substitute in a small bowl.
3. Cut bacon strips in 1/2. Lay them on the sheet pan and dust with the chili powder mixture.
4. Wrap three asparagus spears together with one slice of bacon (with the dusted side facing towards the asparagus); securing each end with a toothpick. You should have 8 packets.
5. Grill uncovered over medium-low heat for 12 minutes turning halfway through or until bacon is crisp.
6. Discard toothpicks and serve immediately. Each serving is 2 wraps.

Nutritional Information
- Protein : 5g
- Fat : 10.2g
- Fiber : 2.4g
- Calories :128

Asparagus, Mushrooms And Peas

Servings: 6 | **Prep:** 15 m | **Style:** American | **Cook**: 25 m

Ingredients
- 3 tbsps Unsalted Butter Stick
- 3 medium (4-1/8" long) Scallions or Spring Onions
- 1 tsp Garlic
- 1 or 3oz Portobello Mushroom Cap
- 1/4 cup Vinegar (Cider)

- 1 cup Tap Water
- 1 lb Asparagus
- 1/2 cup Green Peas
- 2 tbsps Heavy Cream
- 8 leaves Basil
- 1/4 dash Salt
- 1/4 tsp Black Pepper

Directions
1. In a large skillet, melt 2 tablespoons butter over medium-high heat. Reduce heat to medium. Add scallions, and cook until green portion is wilted, about 3 minutes.
2. Add garlic (minced), and cook for 30 seconds.
3. Add remaining tablespoon butter; when melted, add mushrooms. Cook, stirring occasionally, until mushrooms are softened, about 5 minutes.
4. Add vinegar, and cook for 2 minutes.
5. Pour the water into skillet. Add asparagus, and bring to boil over medium-high heat. Reduce heat to medium, and simmer for 5 minutes.
6. Add peas, and cook for 2 minutes.
7. Add heavy cream, and continue to simmer until sauce thickens, about 2 minutes.
8. Transfer to a serving bowl, stir in basil, and season to taste with salt and pepper.
9. Sprinkle with Parmesan, if desired. Serve immediately.

Nutritional Information
- Protein : 3g
- Fat : 7.8g
- Fiber : 2.6g
- Calories :103

Atkins Chocolate Slushies

Servings: 4 | **Prep:** 120 m | **Style:** American | **Cook:** 10 m

Ingredients
- 1 cup Heavy Cream
- 1/2 cup Tap Water
- 2 tbsps Cocoa Powder (Unsweetened)
- 8 tbsps Sugar Free Chocolate Syrup
- 1 tsp Vanilla Extract

Directions
1. In a medium saucepan combine cream, water, cocoa powder and 1/2 cup unsweetened chocolate syrup.
2. Bring to a boil over medium heat. Reduce heat to low; cook, stirring occasionally, 5 minutes. Remove from heat and stir in vanilla.
3. Pour mixture into two ice cube trays. Freeze 2 hours.
4. Before serving transfer cubes into a food processor. Pulse until mixture is finely chopped and slushy.

Nutritional Information
- Protein : 1.8g
- Fat : 22.6g
- Fiber : 0.9g
- Calories :216

Atkins Cinnamon Pie Crust

Servings: 8 | **Prep:** 10 m | **Style:** American

Ingredients
- 1/4 tsp Salt
- 1 tsp Sucralose Based Sweetener (Sugar Substitute)
- 1 tsp Cinnamon
- 1/2 cup Unsalted Butter Stick
- 3 3/4 servings All Purpose Low-Carb Baking Mix
- 2 tbsps Tap Water

Directions

Use the Atkins recipe to make All Purpose Low-Carb Baking Mix. You will need 1 1/4 cups to make one pie crust.

1. Pulse the baking mix, salt, sugar substitute, and cinnamon in a food processor to incorporate; add butter and pulse until mixture resembles a coarse meal, about 30 seconds. Pulse in water until dough just comes together, about 30 seconds (add up to 1 more tablespoon if necessary).
2. Transfer dough to a sheet of plastic wrap; form into a a disk about 6 inches in diameter. Wrap tightly in plastic; refrigerate until firm, about 30 minutes.
3. Roll and bake as directed in pie recipe. Makes 1 pie crust.

Nutritional Information
- Protein : 14.8g
- Fat : 13.6g
- Fiber : 1.7g

- Calories :193

Atkins Coconut Layer Cake

Servings: 12 | **Prep**: 30 m | **Style**: American | **Cook**: 22 m

Ingredients
- large Eggs (Whole)
- 1 1/2 cups Sucralose Based Sweetener (Sugar Substitute)
- 3 tsps Coconut Extract
- 2/3 cup Whole Grain Soy Flour
- 1 tsp Baking Powder (Straight Phosphate, Double Acting)
- 6 large Egg Whites
- 2 cups Unsalted Butter Stick
- 1/4 tsp Salt
- 2/3 cup Dried Coconut

Directions
1. Heat oven to 350°F. Grease two 8-inch cake pans; line bottoms with parchment paper; then grease the paper. Melt 1/2 cup butter and set aside. Place remaining butter (1 1/2 cups) on a plate, cut it into 1 Tbsp portions, and keep it at room temperature.
2. With an electric mixer on high, beat whole eggs, 3/4 cup sugar substitute and 1 tbsp coconut extract until ribbons form, about 5 minutes.
3. In three additions cup sift soy flour, baking power and salt over egg mixture; fold in with a rubber spatula to combine.
4. Fold in 1/2 cup melted butter. Then pour batter into prepared pans.

5. Bake for 22 minutes until cake springs back in middle when lightly touched. Cool in pans on wire racks 5 minutes. Line racks with paper towels and invert cake layers. Gently peel off parchment and cool completely.
6. For frosting: in a double boiler or a bowl placed over simmering water, whisk egg whites, 3/4 cup sugar substitute and salt until temperature reaches 130°F. Transfer whites to mixing bowl and beat on high speed until cool and fully whipped. Reduce speed to medium and beat in 1 1/2 cups room temperature butter 1 tablespoon at a time until well combined, thick and creamy, about 10 minutes - do not rush the process.
7. Place one cake layer on serving plate. Mix 1 cup frosting with half the coconut (1/3 cup); frost bottom layer. Place top cake layer over bottom layer. Cover top and sides with remaining frosting and pat remaining 1/3 cup coconut over frosting. Optional: toast coconut (3-5 minutes at 350°F). Makes 12 servings.

Nutritional Information
- Protein : 8g
- Fat : 38g
- Fiber : 1g
- Calories :397

Atkins Cuisine Brownies

Servings: 25 | **Prep:** 15 m | **Style:** American | **Cook:** 30 m

Ingredients
- 4 oz Unsweetened Baking Chocolate Squares
- 1/2 cup Unsalted Butter Stick
- 1/2 cup Heavy Cream

- 5 large Eggs (Whole)
- 1 cup Sucralose Based Sweetener (Sugar Substitute)
- 2 tsps Baking Powder (Straight Phosphate, Double Acting)
- 4 1/2 servings All Purpose Low-Carb Baking Mix

Directions
1. Use the Atkins recipe to make All Purpose Low-Carb Baking Mix to use in this recipe. You will need 1 1/4 cups.
2. Pre-heat oven to 325°F.
3. Place the unsweetened chocolate and butter together in a bowl and microwave on high power for approximately 2 minutes until chocolate is melted. Whisk in heavy cream.
4. In a separate bowl, add the eggs and 1 cup of granular sugar substitute. Beat together using an electric mixer until mixture is just blended. Reduce mixer to low speed and then blend in the chocolate mixture.
5. With a wooden spoon, mix in the baking powder and 1 1/4 cups low-carb baking mix.
6. Coat 8 x 8 inch pan with non-stick vegetable oil spray and spread batter evenly into pan.
7. Bake at 325°F for 30-35 minutes or until done (toothpick inserted in the center comes out clean). (Do not over-bake or brownies will be dry and hard.)
8. Once cooled, cut into 5 rows by 5 rows to make 25 brownies.

Nutritional Information
- Protein : 6.6g
- Fat : 9.4g
- Fiber : 1.2g
- Calories :119

Atkins Cuisine Cookies

Servings: 36 | **Prep:** 20 m | **Style:** American | **Cook:** 10 m

Ingredients
- 1 tsp Baking Powder (Straight Phosphate, Double Acting)
- 1/2 tsp Salt
- 1 cup Salted Butter Stick
- 1 cup Sucralose Based Sweetener (Sugar Substitute)
- 2 tsps Vanilla Extract
- 2 large Eggs (Whole)
- 6 servings All Purpose Low-Carb Baking Mix
- 6 oz Sugar Free Chocolate Chips

Directions

Use the Atkins recipe to make All Purpose Low-Carb Baking Mix for this recipe; you will need 2 cups but the recipe makes 3. Save any remaining in an airtight container in the refrigerator.

1. Preheat oven to 375°F.
2. Blend all dry ingredients together in a small mixing bowl, set aside.
3. Mix melted butter, sugar substitute and vanilla at medium speed with an electric mixer until well blended. Add eggs one at a time, mixing well after each addition. Gradually add dry ingredient mixture, beating until blended. Gently mix in chocolate chips with a wooden spoon or spatula.
4. Spoon rounded teaspoonfuls of cookie dough onto a cookie sheet coated with non-stick vegetable oil spray. Gently flatten cookies by pressing with hand or spatula.
5. Cook at 375° F for 10 to 12 minutes or until done or until lightly browned. Remove from baking sheet and place

cookies on a wire rack to cool. (Do not overbake cookies or they will be dry and hard.)

Nutritional Information
- Protein : 6.65.7g
- Fat : 7.7g
- Fiber : 0.8g
- Calories :103

Atkins Cuisine Pizza With Sausage, Bell Peppers And Onions

Servings: 8 | **Prep:** 20 m | **Style:** American | **Cook**: 30 m

Ingredients
- 1 1/2 tsps Baking Powder (Straight Phosphate, Double Acting)
- 1/2 tsp Salt
- 1 individual packet Sucralose Based Sweetener (Sugar Substitute)
- 1 cup Tap Water
- 3 tbsps Extra Virgin Olive Oil
- 1/2 cup Tomato Sauce
- 1 cup shredded Whole Milk Mozzarella Cheese
- 1 link (5" long) Italian Sausage
- 1/2 medium (approx 2-3/4" long, 2-1/2" dia) Green Sweet Pepper
- 1/2 medium (approx 2-3/4" long, 2-1/2" dia) Red Sweet Pepper
- 1 small Red Onion
- 6 servings All Purpose Low-Carb Baking Mix

Directions

Use the Atkins recipe to make All Purpose Low-Carb Baking Mix for this recipe. You will need 2 cups.

1. Preheat oven to 425°F.
2. Blend together baking mix, baking powder, salt and sugar substitute in a large mixing bowl.
3. Add water and oil. Using a wooden spoon or a spatula, combine into a dough. Using a spatula, remove the dough from the bowl and place on a clean surface lightly coated with olive oil spray.
4. Coat rolling pin with oil spray and roll the dough out to fit the pizza pan or stone. Or use your hands to pat the dough into shape.
5. Bake the crust for 10 minutes and remove from oven.
6. Spread tomato sauce evenly over the pizza. Sprinkle with mozzarella and top with sausage rounds, green and red bell pepper slices and onions. Sprinkle with salt and pepper to taste.
7. Return to the oven and continue baking for 10-15 minutes. Cut into 8 slices.

Nutritional Information
- Protein : 28.6g
- Fat : 15.3g
- Fiber : 3g
- Calories :282

Atkins Cuisine Pizza-Barbecue Chicken Supreme

Servings: 8 | **Prep:** 20 m | **Style:** American | **Cook:** 30 m

Ingredients
- 1 1/2 tsps Baking Powder (Straight Phosphate, Double Acting)
- 1/2 tsp Salt
- 1 individual packet Sucralose Based Sweetener (Sugar Substitute)
- 1 cup Tap Water
- 1 small Red Onion
- 1 cup cooked, diced Chicken Breast
- 2 servings Barbecue Sauce
- 1/2 medium (approx 2-3/4" long, 2-1/2" dia) Green Sweet Pepper
- 6 servings All Purpose Low-Carb Baking Mix
- 1 cup shredded Whole Milk Mozzarella Cheese
- 3 tbsps Extra Virgin Olive Oil

Directions

Using barbecue sauce instead of tomato sauce spices up the chicken topping. You can substitute other vegetable and meat toppings for variety.

1. Heat oven to 425°F.
2. Blend together baking mix (2 cups), baking powder, salt and sugar substitute in a large mixing bowl.
3. Add water and oil. Using a wooden spoon or a spatula, combine into a dough. Using a spatula, remove the dough

from the bowl and place on a clean surface lightly coated with olive oil spray.
4. Coat rolling pin with oil spray and roll the dough out to fit the pizza pan or stone. Or use your hands to pat the dough into shape.
5. Bake the crust for 10 minutes and remove from oven.
6. Spread Barbecue Sauce (about 1/2 cup) evenly over the pizza. Sprinkle with mozzarella and top with chicken pieces, bell pepper slices and onions. Sprinkle with salt and pepper, to taste.
7. Return to the oven and continue baking for 10-15 minutes. Cut into 8 slices.

Nutritional Information
- Protein : 27.3g
- Fat : 13.3g
- Fiber : 4.9g
- Calories :263

Atkins Yorkshire Pudding

Servings: 9 | **Prep**: 5 m | **Style:** Other | **Cook:** 35 m

Ingredients
- 1/2 cup Whole Grain Soy Flour
- 2 oz Vital Wheat Gluten
- 3 large Eggs (Whole)
- 1 cup Whole Milk
- 1 tsp Salt
- 1/3 cup Canola Vegetable Oil
- 1 tsp Baking Powder (Straight Phosphate, Double Acting)

Directions
1. Preheat oven to 450° F.
2. Whisk together soy flour, gluten, eggs, milk and salt.
3. Pour drippings or oil into an 8-inch square baking dish, and place on center rack in oven for 5 minutes, until drippings or oil is smoking hot. Then add batter and bake 15 minutes.
4. Lower temperature to 350° F and bake for 15 to 20 minutes more, until lightly browned. Serve piping hot.

Nutritional Information
- Protein : 9.2g
- Fat : 11.8g
- Fiber : 0.5g
- Calories :157

Avocado Gazpacho Smoothie

Servings: **1** | Prep: **5 m** | Style: **Mexican**

Ingredients
- 1 cup Tap Water
- 1 fruit without skin and seed California Avocado
- 1 oz Goat Cheese (Soft)
- 1 tbsp Heavy Cream
- 2 tsp choppeds Chives
- 2 tsps Fresh Lime Juice
- 1/8 tsp Salt

Directions
1. Place cut-up avocado in a blender. Add remaining ingredients, and blend until smooth. If needed, add additional water, 1 tablespoon at a time, to reach desired consistency.
2. Pour into a tall glass, and garnish with chives and an avocado slice, if desired. Serve immediately.

Nutritional Information
- Protein : 9.2g
- Fat : 35g
- Fiber : 9.3g
- Calories :385

Avocado Zucchini Soup

Servings: 4 | **Prep:** 10 m | **Style:** American | **Cook:** 15 m

Ingredients
- 1 fruit without skin and seed California Avocado
- 2 tbsps Extra Virgin Olive Oil
- 4 medium (4-1/8" long) Scallions or Spring Onions
- 1 tsp Ginger
- 1 clove Garlic
- 2 medium Zucchinis
- 29 oz Bouillon Vegetable Broth
- 1 cup Tap Water
- 1/2 tsp Salt

- 1/2 tsp Black Pepper
- 1 tbsp Fresh Lemon Juice
- 1/16 cup chopped Sweet Red Peppers

Directions
1. Heat oil in a large saucepan over medium heat. Add 2/3 of the green onions and cook 3 minutes; stir in ginger and garlic and cook, stirring, 1 minute more. Add broth, water, zucchini, salt, and pepper.
2. Cover and cook 10 minutes, until zucchini is very soft. Cool slightly. Then, stir in avocado.
3. Puree soup in batches in a food processor or blender. Return to pan to heat through and stir in lemon juice.
4. Garnish with red pepper and remaining green onions.

Nutritional Information
- Protein : 2.4g
- Fat : 12.6g
- Fiber : 4g
- Calories :156

Baby Greens With Grapefruit And Red Onion

Servings: 4 | **Prep:** 15 m | **Style:** Mexican

Ingredients
- 1 fruit (3-3/4" dia) Grapefruit (Pink and Red)
- 1 fruit (3-3/4" dia) White Grapefruit
- 1/4 tsp Yellow Mustard Seed

- 3 tbsps Extra Virgin Olive Oil
- 1 tsp Tarragon
- 3 3/4 cups Spring Mix Salad
- 1/2 small Red Onion

Directions

If you don't have a grapefruit knife to easily remove the segments, use this method: Slice off just enough of the top and bottom of each grapefruit so they can stand upright on a cutting board. Using a sharp chefs knife and working from the top, circle the entire fruit, peeling the skin off and leaving very little of the bitter white pith behind. Using a smaller paring knife, cut out each segment from the white membrane. Squeeze out any remaining juice from fruit when done. Reserve 1 tablespoon of juice for the dressing and save the additional juice for another use.

1. Section grapefruits.
2. Add reserved grapefruit juice to a mixing bowl. Add mustard. Slowly drizzle in olive oil, whisking well, until well combined.
3. Stir in tarragon; add salt and freshly ground black pepper to taste, set aside.
4. Add greens and toss gently with grapefruit sections, red onion and salad dressing.

Nutritional Information

- Protein : 1.9g
- Fat : 10.7g
- Fiber : 3.1g
- Calories :149

Baby Spinach, Pickled Beets And Tomato Salad

Servings: 1 | **Prep:** 5 m | **Style:** American

Ingredients
- 1 1/2 cups Baby Spinach
- 1/4 cup sliced Pickled Beets
- 5 Cherry Tomatoes

Directions
1. Place the spinach leaves in a bowl. Add beets and tomatoes and gently toss with low-carb salad dressing of your choice.
2. Season to taste with salt and freshly ground black pepper.

Nutritional Information
- Protein : 2.2g
- Fat : 0.2g
- Fiber : 3.5g
- Calories :57

Bacon And Goat Cheese Salad

Servings: 6 | **Prep:** 25 m | **Style:** Other | **Cook:** 15 m

Ingredients
- 2 cups chopped Endive
- 3 tbsps chopped Chives
- 8 oz Goat Cheese (Soft)
- 2 tbsps Extra Virgin Olive Oil
- 1 large Egg (Whole)
- 1 1/2 tbsps Red Wine Vinegar
- 1 tbsp Dijon Mustard
- 1 1/2 servings Atkins Cuisine Bread
- 3/4 tsp Black Pepper
- 4 cups shredded Cos or Romaine Lettuce
- 6 medium slice (yield after cooking) Bacon

Directions
1. FOR SALAD: Cook bacon in a large nonstick skillet over medium heat, turning once, until crisp, about 6 to 7 minutes. Transfer with a slotted spoon to paper towels. Reserve 1 tablespoon of bacon drippings.
2. In a large bowl, combine romaine, endive, and chives; set aside.
3. In a food processor or blender, process bread to make crumbs; spread crumbs on a plate. Place goat cheese slices cut side down on work surface and press lightly to flatten. Dip each slice in egg; let excess drip off. Place on crumbs, pressing to coat evenly and completely.
4. Wipe out bacon skillet with a paper towel; add oil and heat over medium heat. Add goat-cheese patties and cook until browned, about 2 minutes per side (reduce heat if browning

occurs too fast or cheese is melting). Transfer to a plate lined with paper towels. Remove skillet from heat.
5. DRESSING: Add reserved bacon drippings, olive oil, vinegar, mustard and pepper to skillet. Whisk to combine. Add warm dressing and bacon to bowl with greens. Toss to combine. Arrange salad on individual serving plates and top each with a goat-cheese patty.

Nutritional Information
- Protein : 13.8g
- Fat : 27.8g
- Fiber : 1.7g
- Calories :320

Bacon Wrapped Filet With Blue Cheese Butter Sauce

Servings: 2 | **Style:** American | **Cook:** 45 m

Ingredients
- 2 medium (4-1/8" long) Young Green Onions
- 4 oz Portobello Mushroom Cap
- 3 Cherry Tomatoes
- 12 oz Beef Tenderloin (Lean Only, Trimmed to 1/8" Fat)
- 2 slices Bacon
- 1 tbsp Unsalted Butter Stick
- 3 oz Blue Cheese
- 1/3 tbsp Red Wine Vinegar
- 8 oz Baby Spinach
- 2 tsps Olive Oil

- 1/4 tsp Salt
- 1/4 tsp Black Pepper

Directions
1. Preheat the oven to 425ºF. Finely dice the green part of the green onions and place in a small bowl. Dice the white part of the onion and set aside. Remove the cap from the mushroom and discard the stem. Chop the mushroom into ¼-inch pieces; set aside.
2. Pat dry the beef with paper towels. Slice the tenderloin in half widthwise and press down on the halves slightly into filet mignon steaks. Season each filet with ⅛ teaspoon each of salt and pepper. Wrap the outer edge of each steak with a bacon slice. Set aside.
3. Add the butter and 1 ounce of the blue cheese to the bowl with the green onions and stir until well combined. Pour the red wine vinegar into another small bowl, add ¼ teaspoon each of salt and pepper and slowly whisk in 1 tablespoon of olive oil; hold.
4. Heat 2 teaspoons of olive oil in a large non-stick sauté pan over medium-high heat. When the oil is hot, add the steaks and sear on all sides, turning frequently with tongs until browned, about 3 minutes. Transfer to a sheet pan lined with foil and roast for 6 to 8 minutes, or until desired doneness.
5. Meanwhile, in the same sauté pan over medium-high heat, add the mushrooms and the white part of the onion, season with ⅛ teaspoon each of salt and pepper and reduce the heat to low. Saute while stirring until the mushrooms are tender, about 4 minutes. Place the baby spinach in a large bowl and add the remaining 2 ounces of blue cheese. Drizzle the vinaigrette over the spinach. Toss until well combined.
6. Spoon the mushrooms evenly onto two plates. Top with a filet and a dollop of the blue cheese butter. Arrange the salad next to steak and enjoy!

Nutritional Information
- Protein : 54.5g
- Fat : 36.2g
- Fiber : 4g
- Calories :581

Bacon-Egg Salad Flatout Wrap

Servings: 1 | **Prep**: 10 m | **Style:** American

Ingredients
- 2 large Boiled Eggs
- 1 tbsp Real Mayonnaise
- 1/2 tsp or 1 packet Yellow Mustard
- 1 flatbread Light Original Flatbread
- 1 1/2 oz cooked Turkey Bacon

Directions
1. Mix together chopped eggs, mayonnaise and mustard. Add salt and pepper to taste.
2. Spread mixture on one rounded end of Flatout. Top with cooked crumbled bacon.
3. Roll up and cut in half.

Nutritional Information
- Protein : 34.4g
- Fat : 36.1g
- Fiber : 10.2g
- Calories :511

Bahian Halibut

Servings: 4 | **Prep:** 10 m | **Style:** Other | **Cook:** 10 m

Ingredients
- 2 tbsps Extra Virgin Olive Oil
- 2 tbsps Fresh Lime Juice
- 2 lbs Atlantic and Pacific Halibut
- 4 tbsps chopped Onions
- 1 cup chopped Green Sweet Pepper
- 1 pepper Serrano Pepper
- 1 tsp Garlic
- 1 tsp Salt
- 1/2 cup Coconut Cream
- 1 small whole (2-2/5" dia) Red Tomato

Directions
1. The state of Bahia in Brazil borders the Caribbean and includes what is known as the Coconut Coast and was first settled by the Portuguese. This heat of this well-seasoned fish dish is tamed with coconut milk.
2. With a fork, whisk 1 tablespoon oil and all the lime juice on large platter, add fish, and turn to coat. Dice the onion, bell pepper and the serrano pepper (be sure to use gloves to protect your hands from the heat of the pepper - do not include the seeds or ribs if you want to reduce the heat). Mince the garlic and add to a bowl with the onions and peppers. Chop the tomatoes, place in a small bowl and set aside.
3. Heat remaining tablespoon oil in a 12-inch nonstick skillet over medium heat. Add garlic and the diced onion and peppers. Cook 6 minutes until onion is translucent and peppers are just tender.

4. Sprinkle 1/2 teaspoon of salt over fish and add fish to skillet; pour coconut milk over fish and add tomato. Reduce heat to medium-low and simmer 8 to 9 minutes, turning fish halfway through cooking time.
5. Stir remaining salt into sauce, spoon over fish a few times, and serve immediately.

Nutritional Information
- Protein : 48.6g
- Fat : 19.5g
- Fiber : 1.8g
- Calories :400

Baked Artichoke-Parsley Cheese Squares

Servings: 8 | **Prep:** 10 m | **Style:** American | **Cook:** 35 m

Ingredients
- 2 tbsps Extra Virgin Olive Oil
- 3 medium (4-1/8" long) Scallions or Spring Onions
- 3 tsps Garlic
- 1 package (9 oz) Artichokes (Globe or French, Unprepared, Frozen)
- 1/2 tsp Oregano
- 1/4 tsp Crushed Red Pepper Flakes
- 4 large Eggs (Whole)
- 1 cup shredded Monterey Jack Cheese
- 1/8 cup dry Whole Grain Soy Flour
- 2 tbsps Parsley
- 1/2 tsp Salt
- 1/4 tsp Black Pepper

Directions
1. Preheat oven to 325°F.
2. In a medium skillet over medium-high heat, heat oil and sauté green onion until softened, about 4 minutes. Add garlic and sauté until aroma is released, about 30 seconds. Add artichokes, oregano and pepper flakes and cook until artichokes are warmed through, about 2 minutes. Allow to cool slightly, about 5 minutes.
3. In a large bowl, gently whisk eggs, cheese, soy flour, parsley, salt and pepper until well-combined. Using a wooden spoon, stir in artichoke mixture.
4. Pour artichoke batter into an 8 square baking dish and bake 30 minutes, until set and slightly golden on top. Cool slightly before cutting into squares.

Nutritional Information
- Protein : 11.6g
- Fat : 14.8g

Baked Catfish With Broccoli And Herb-Butter Blend

Servings: 1 | **Prep:** 5 m | **Style:** American | **Cook:** 15 m

Ingredients
- 6 oz Channel Catfish (Farmed)
- 1 cup chopped Broccoli
- 1 serving Herb-Butter Blend

Directions
1. Cooking fish in an aluminum-foil packet makes for easy cleanup and works especially well for single portions. Add a vegetable and you have a complete quick meal. Use any compound butter or use 1 tablespoon of the Atkins recipe: Herb-Butter Blend.
2. Preheat oven to 350°F.
3. Place the catfish on a 12-inch square piece of foil. Sprinkle fish with salt and freshly ground pepper to taste. Arrange broccoli florets around fish.
4. Fold up the sides of the foil and crimp tightly to form a sealed packet.
5. Bake for 10 15 minutes until fish is flaky and broccoli is tender.
6. Transfer to a dish, open foil and top with a tablespoon of Herb-Butter Blend.

Nutritional Information
- Protein : 28.7g
- Fat : 25.9g
- Fiber : 2.2g
- Calories :362

Baked Chicken With Artichokes

Servings: 4 | **Prep:** 20 m | **Style**: American | **Cook:** 40 m

Ingredients
- 8 oz Mushroom Pieces and Stems
- 1/2 tsp Salt
- 1/2 cup chopped Onions
- 20 oz boneless (yield after cooking) Chicken Thigh

- 4 1/2 tsps Garlic
- 4 fl ozs Sauvignon Blanc Wine
- 1 tsp Rosemary
- 1/4 tsp Crushed Red Pepper Flakes
- 1 1/2 tsp grounds Oregano
- 3 tbsps Extra Virgin Olive Oil
- 1 package (9 oz), yield Artichokes (Globe or French) (with Salt, Frozen, Drained, Cooked, Boiled)
- 1/2 tsp Black Pepper
- 3/4 serving All Purpose Low-Carb Baking Mix

Directions
1. Use the Atkins recipe to make All Purpose Low-Carb Baking Mix for this recipe. Dredging chicken in flour before sautéing seals in the juices and give it a nice color.
2. Preheat oven to 350°F. Place 1/4 cup baking mix, salt and pepper in a shallow plate and mix well. Dredge chicken in the mixture, turning to coat evenly and then tapping to remove any excess.
3. In large skillet, heat oil over medium-high heat. Cook chicken until lightly browned, turning once, about 4 minutes. Transfer to baking dish.
4. Add onion to skillet and sauté until softened, about 2 minutes. Add mushrooms and sauté until lightly golden, about 3 more minutes. Add garlic and sauté until aroma is released, about 30 seconds. Stir in wine, artichokes, rosemary and red pepper flakes and bring to a simmer.
5. Pour artichoke mixture over chicken in the baking dish, cover and bake 40 minutes, until chicken is tender and cooked through. Season with additional salt and pepper, if desired, and stir in oregano before serving.

Nutritional Information

- Protein : 37.5g
- Fat : 17.8g
- Fiber : 4.9g
- Calories :376

Baked Fennel Au Gratin

Servings: 6 | **Prep:** 5 m | **Style:** French | **Cook:** 50 m

Ingredients
- 2 bulbs Fennel Bulk
- 1/2 tsp Salt
- 1/4 tsp Black Pepper
- 1 cup Heavy Cream
- 1/2 cup shredded Gruyere Cheese
- 2 tbsps Parmesan Cheese (Grated)
- 1/2 serving All Purpose Low-Carb Baking Mix
- 1/4 cup Unsalted Butter Stick

Directions
1. Use the Atkins recipe to make All Purpose Low-Carb Baking Mix for this recipe.
2. Preheat oven to 375°F.
3. Grease a shallow 2-quart baking dish with 1 teaspoon butter and set aside.
4. Trim fennel leaving 1 stalks, Quarter bulbs and remove center core. Cut crosswise into 1/4 slices. Place fennel in a saucepan and cook in lightly salted water over medium heat until just tender, about 10 minutes. Drain fennel and season with salt and pepper. Transfer fennel to dish, pressing down to form an even layer. Set aside.

5. In a medium saucepan melt butter over medium heat. Stir in 3 Tbsp baking mix and cook 2 minutes.
6. Add cream and bring to a boil. Cook, whisking constantly, until slightly, about 5 minutes. Turn off heat and stir in Gruyere until melted.
7. Pour sauce evenly over fennel and sprinkle dish with Parmesan cheese. Cover with foil and bake 15 minutes; uncover and bake 15-20 minutes more until golden brown and bubbly.

Nutritional Information
- Protein : 8.1g
- Fat : 26.4g
- Fiber : 2.7g
- Calories :293

Baked Goat Cheese And Ricotta Custards

Servings: 4 | **Style:** Italian | **Cook:** 50 m

Ingredients
- 1 1/3 second sprays Original Canola Cooking Spray
- 1 cup Ricotta Cheese (Whole Milk)
- 6 oz Goats Cheese (Semisoft)
- 3 tbsps Parmesan Cheese (Grated)
- 1/4 cup chopped English Walnuts
- 12 leaves Spinach
- 2 large Eggs (Whole)
- 1/8 tsp Salt
- 1/8 tsp Black Pepper
- 2 tbsps Basil

Directions
1. Heat oven to 350°F. Spray cooking spray onto four 5-ounce ramekins or custard cups.
2. Combine ricotta, goat cheese, Parmesan, walnuts, basil, egg, salt, and pepper in a bowl and mix well.
3. Line each ramekin with 3 spinach leaves. Divide cheese mixture; fill full. Bake 30 minutes. Cool 5 minutes.
4. To serve, run a knife around the rim of each custard. Invert onto small plates. Salt and pepper to taste.

Nutritional Information
- Protein : 22.3g
- Fat : 28g
- Fiber : 1.1g
- Calories :360

Baked Meatballs

Servings: 4 | **Prep:** 8 m | **Style:** American | **Cook:** 35 m

Ingredients
- 1 tbsp Extra Virgin Olive Oil
- 1/2 large Scallions or Spring Onion
- 1 1/2 tsps Garlic
- 1/2 lb Ground Veal
- 1/2 lb Ground Beef (80% Lean / 20% Fat)
- 1/2 lb Ground Pork
- 1/2 cup Parmesan Cheese (Grated)
- 2 large Eggs (Whole)
- 1/2 tsp Salt

- 1/4 tsp Black Pepper

Directions

If possible, have the butcher grind together the three different meats. Be sure to wash your hands thoroughly after handling raw pork.

1. Heat oven to 375°F.
2. In a skillet, over high heat, heat oil, cook onion 5 minutes, stirring frequently, until softened. Add garlic (minced) and cook 1 minute more.
3. Transfer to a bowl and mix in ground meats, cheese, eggs, salt, and pepper. Roll into golf ball-size meatballs. Place on a jelly roll pan.
4. Bake 20- 25 minutes, until browned and cooked through.

Nutritional Information
- Protein : 38.6g
- Fat : 26.7g
- Fiber : 0.2g
- Calories :409

Baked Quesadillas

Servings: 4 | **Prep:** 10 m | **Style:** Mexican | **Cook:** 10 m

Ingredients
- 2 tbsps Light Olive Oil
- 2 tbsps chopped Onions

- 16 oz Pork Chops or Roasts (Center Rib, Bone-In)
- 8 slice (1 oz) Monterey Jack Cheese
- 1/4 cup Green Tomato Chile Sauce (Salsa Verde)
- 1 Jalapeno Pepper
- 1/4 cup Cilantro (Coriander)
- 1/2 tsp Black Pepper
- 1/4 tsp Salt
- 1 tortilla Low Carb Tortillas

Directions
1. Make sure the tortillas contain no more than 3 grams of Net Carbs each. Serve with sour cream and additional red or green salsa, if desired.
2. Heat oven to 450°F.
3. Heat 1 tablespoon of the oil in large skillet over medium-high heat. Cook chopped white onion 5 minutes, until softened.
4. Transfer to a bowl. Add pork, cheese, green salsa, chopped jalapeño, cilantro, pepper and salt. Mix well.
5. Brush one side of each tortilla with remaining oil.
6. Spoon one-sixth of pork mixture over half of non-oiled side of each tortilla and fold in half over filling.
7. Place on a baking sheet. Bake 5 minutes, until crisp and golden.

Nutritional Information
- Protein : 43.4g
- Fat : 40.3g
- Fiber : 1g
- Calories :569

Baked Red Bell Peppers Filled With Cherry Tomatoes And Feta

Servings: 4 | **Prep:** 10 m | **Style:** American | **Cook:** 45 m

Ingredients
- 2 medium (approx 2-3/4" long, 2-1/2" dia) Sweet Red Peppers
- 2 oz Feta Cheese
- 8 Cherry Tomatoes
- 1/2 tsp ground Thyme (Dried)
- 2 tbsps Basil
- 1 tbsp Extra Virgin Olive Oil

Directions
1. Preheat oven to 400°F.
2. Cut peppers in half lengthwise. Remove stems, ribs and seeds.
3. Gently combine feta, tomatoes, thyme and basil. Fill pepper halves with the mixture.
4. Place in a baking dish and drizzle with olive oil.
5. Bake, covered with aluminum foil, for 30 minutes. Remove foil and bake an additional 15 minutes until the tomatoes burst and cheese is golden-brown.

Nutritional Information
- Protein : 3.2g
- Fat : 6.8g
- Fiber : 1.9g

- Calories :97

Baked Salmon With Bok Choy And Mixed Greens

Servings: 1 | **Prep:** 15 m | **Style:** American | **Cook:** 10 m

Ingredients
- 3/4 cup chopped Snowpeas (Pea Pod)
- 1/16 tsp Salt
- 8 oz Chinese Cabbage (Bok-Choy, Pak-Choi)
- 2 oz Pickled Okra
- 3 oz Cooked Red Peppers
- 1/16 tsp Black Pepper
- 1/2 oz Salsa
- 1/2 tbsp Extra Virgin Olive Oil
- 1 tbsp Reserva Sherry Vinegar
- 1/4 tbsp Unsalted Butter Stick
- 6 oz Atlantic Salmon (Farmed)
- 1 cup shredded or chopped Mixed Salad Greens

Directions
1. Use the Atkins recipe for Sherry Vinaigrette for the salad.
2. Preheat oven to 475° F. Place olive oil and butter in a skillet large enough to hold fish in a single layer.
3. Place skillet with just the olive oil and butter into the oven for 3 minutes, until butter is melted. Season fish with salt and pepper. Place fish flesh side down in prepared skillet. Bake 10 minutes, turning carefully once halfway through cooking time, until just cooked through.

4. Remove from skillet; tent with foil. Add bok choy and lemon peel to skillet. Stir to coat with pan's oil. Place in oven 1 minute, until leaves are wilted and stems are warmed through.
5. To make puree, blend peppers and salsa in a blender 30 seconds.
6. Top bok choy with fish and dollop with the purée.
7. Toss the greens, okra, peppers and snow peas with the Sherry Vinaigrette. Serve with the salmon and bok choy.

Nutritional Information
- Protein : 37.5g
- Fat : 44.1g
- Fiber : 7.9g
- Calories :623

Baked Salmon With Bok Choy And Red Bell Pepper Purée

Servings: 4 | **Prep:** 10 m | **Style:** American | **Cook:** 10 m

Ingredients
- 3/4 cup chopped Snowpeas (Pea Pod)
- 1/16 tsp Salt
- 8 oz Chinese Cabbage (Bok-Choy, Pak-Choi)
- 2 oz Pickled Okra
- 3 oz Cooked Red Peppers
- 1/16 tsp Black Pepper
- 1/2 oz Salsa

- 1/2 tbsp Extra Virgin Olive Oil
- 1 tbsp Reserva Sherry Vinegar
- 1/4 tbsp Unsalted Butter Stick
- 6 oz Atlantic Salmon (Farmed)
- 1 cup shredded or chopped Mixed Salad Greens

Directions
1. Use the Atkins recipe for Sherry Vinaigrette for the salad.
2. Preheat oven to 475° F. Place olive oil and butter in a skillet large enough to hold fish in a single layer.
3. Place skillet with just the olive oil and butter into the oven for 3 minutes, until butter is melted. Season fish with salt and pepper. Place fish flesh side down in prepared skillet. Bake 10 minutes, turning carefully once halfway through cooking time, until just cooked through.
4. Remove from skillet; tent with foil. Add bok choy and lemon peel to skillet. Stir to coat with pan's oil. Place in oven 1 minute, until leaves are wilted and stems are warmed through.
5. To make puree, blend peppers and salsa in a blender 30 seconds.
6. Top bok choy with fish and dollop with the purée.
7. Toss the greens, okra, peppers and snow peas with the Sherry Vinaigrette. Serve with the salmon and bok choy.

Nutritional Information
- Protein : 31.9g
- Fat : 29.4g
- Fiber : 2g
- Calories :412

Baked Tamari-Lemon Pork Chops

Servings: 4 | **Prep:** 15 m | **Style:** Asian | **Cook:** 40 m

Ingredients
- 8 tbsps Tamari Soybean Sauce
- 2 tbsps Worcestershire Sauce
- 2 tsps Garlic
- 1 fl oz Fresh Lemon Juice
- 1/2 tsp Black Pepper
- 1 tsp Canola Vegetable Oil
- 1 1/2 lbs Pork Chops or Roasts (Center Loin, Bone-In)

Directions
1. If you want to serve a dipping sauce with the chops, rather than boiling the marinade, make a fresh batch.
2. In a shallow dish, combine tamari, Worcestershire sauce, garlic (minced), lemon juice, pepper and oil. Add pork chops and turn to coat evenly.
3. Cover, and refrigerate for at least 1 hour or overnight.
4. Preheat oven to 375°F. Remove chops from marinade and pat dry.
5. Place in a roasting pan and bake for 35 40 minutes.

Nutritional Information
- Protein : 15.2g
- Fat : 8g
- Fiber : 0.1g
- Calories :149

Baked Tofu With Asian Marinade

Servings: 4 | **Prep:** 5 m | **Style:** Asian | **Cook:** 30 m

Ingredients
- 6 oz Firm Silken Tofu
- 1 serving Asian Marinade

Directions
1. Use 2 tablespoons of the Atkins recipe: Asian Marinade.
2. Drain and pat tofu dry with a paper towel. Cut into 1/4 inch strips. Coat with marinade in a shallow dish. Marinate for 30 minutes or more if desired.
3. Preheat oven to 375°
4. Bake on a greased flat pan for 15 minutes, turn over and bake an additional 15 minutes till golden brown and slightly crispy.

Nutritional Information
- Protein : 17.7g
- Fat : 14.9g
- Fiber : 4.8g
- Calories :232

Baked Tofu With Cajun Rub

Servings: 4 | **Prep:** 5 m | **Style:** Asian | **Cook:** 30 m

Ingredients
- 6 oz Firm Silken Tofu
- 1 serving Cajun Rub

- 1 tsp Extra Virgin Olive Oil

Directions
1. Use 1 tablespoon of Atkins recipe: Cajun Rub.
2. Drain and pat tofu dry with a paper towel. Cut into 1/4 inch strips. Rub seasoning and oil onto tofu allow to marinate for 30 minutes if desired. Or rub seasoning into tofu and cook immediately.
3. Preheat oven to 375°
4. Bake on a greased flat pan for 15 minutes, turn over and bake an additional 15 minutes till golden brown and slightly crispy.

Nutritional Information
- Protein : 15.7g
- Fat : 13.6g
- Fiber : 1.9g
- Calories :204

Baked Tofu With Chipotle Marinade

Servings: 1 | **Prep:** 5 m | **Style:** Mexian | **Cook:** 30 m

Ingredients
- 6 oz Firm Silken Tofu
- 1 serving Chipotle Marinade

Directions
1. Use the Atkins recipe to make Chipotle Marinade for this recipe. You will need 2 Tbsp.

2. Drain and pat tofu dry with a paper towel. Cut into 1/4-inch strips. Marinate tofu for 30 minutes (or more if desired) in Chipotle Marinade.
3. Remove from marinade and pat dry. Preheat oven to 375°F.
4. Bake on a greased flat pan for 15 minutes; turn over and bake another 15 minutes until golden brown and slightly crispy.

Nutritional Information
- Protein : 15.8g
- Fat : 15.9g
- Fiber : 1g
- Calories :227

Baked Tofu With Latin Marinade

Servings: 1 | **Prep:** 5 m | **Style:** Mexian | **Cook:** 30 m

Ingredients
- 6 oz Firm Silken Tofu
- 1 serving Latin Marinade

Directions
1. Use 2 tablespoons of the Atkins recipe: Latin Marinade.
2. Drain and pat tofu dry with a paper towel. Cut into 1/4 inch strips and coat with marinade.
3. Preheat oven to 375° 3. Marinate tofu for 30 minutes or more if desired.
4. Bake on a greased flat pan for 15 minutes, turn over and bake an additional 15 minutes till golden brown and slightly crispy. Serve immediately or store in refrigerator for up to 3 days for use on a salad or reheat for a warm dish.

Nutritional Information
- Protein : 15.3g
- Fat : 29.6g
- Fiber : 0.7g
- Calories :344

Baked Tofu With Mediterranean Marinade

Servings: 1 | **Prep:** 5 m | **Style:** Mediterranean / Greek | **Cook:** 30 m

Ingredients
- 6 oz Firm Silken Tofu
- 1 serving Mediterranean Marinade

Directions
1. Drain and pat tofu dry with a paper towel. Cut into 1/4 inch strips.
2. Preheat oven to 375°
3. Marinate tofu in Mediterranean Marinade for 30 minutes or more if desired.
4. Bake on a greased flat pan for 15 minutes, turn over and bake an additional 15 minutes till golden brown and slightly crispy.

Nutritional Information
- Protein : 15.3g

- Fat : 36.7g
- Fiber : 1g
- Calories :405

Baked Tofu With Moroccan Rub

Servings: 1 | **Prep:** 5 m | **Style:** Middle Eastern | **Cook:** 30 m

Ingredients
- 6 oz Firm Silken Tofu
- 1 serving Moroccan Rub
- 1 tsp Extra Virgin Olive Oil

Directions
1. Use the Atkins recipe for Moroccan Rub. You will need 1 Tbsp.
2. Drain and pat tofu dry with a paper towel. Cut into 1/4 inch strips. Rub 1 Tbsp seasoning combined with 1 tsp oil onto tofu allow to marinate for 30 minutes if desired. Or rub seasoning into tofu and cook immediately.
3. Preheat oven to 375°F.
4. Bake on a greased flat pan for 15 minutes, turn over and bake an additional 15 minutes till golden brown and slightly crispy.

Nutritional Information
- Protein : 15.8g
- Fat : 14g
- Fiber : 2.1g
- Calories :210

Baked Tofu With Red Bell Pepper, Broccoli And Peanut Sauce

Servings: 4 | **Prep:** 10 m | **Style:** American | **Cook:** 22 m

Ingredients
- 28 oz Firm Silken Tofu
- 2 tbsps Canola Vegetable Oil
- 3 tbsps Soy Sauce Tamari
- 2 medium (approx 2-3/4" long, 2-1/2" dia) Sweet Red Peppers
- 2 cups chopped Broccoli
- 4 tbsps Natural Creamy Peanut Butter 1/3 Less Sodium & Sugar
- 1 1/2 fl ozs Lime Juice
- 3 tsps Chili Garlic Sauce
- 2 tsps Sucralose Based Sweetener (Sugar Substitute)
- 1/4 cup Cilantro (Coriander)

Directions
1. Preheat oven to 450°.
2. Combine 2 Tbsp tamari soy sauce and 2 Tbsp oil, set aside.
3. Cut tofu into 6 rectangles, brush with soy and oil mixture. Place on baking pan.
4. Add peppers and broccoli to baking pan and brush with soy and oil mixture. Bake for 10 minutes, turn tofu pieces over and continue to bake for an additional 12 minutes till tofu is browned and vegetables are softened.
5. While tofu and vegetable are baking, combine, peanut butter, lime juice, 1 Tbsp tamari, chili garlic sauce and sugar

substitute in a sauce pan over low heat until warmed through.
6. Toss baked tofu and vegetables with sauce and serve immediately with cilantro on top.

Nutritional Information
- Protein : 24.4g
- Fat : 25.7g
- Fiber : 4g
- Calories :377

Balsamic Pork Loin And Cauliflower

Servings: 2 | **Prep:** m | **Style:** American | **Cook:** 45 m

Ingredients
- 28 oz Firm Silken Tofu
- 2 tbsps Canola Vegetable Oil
- 3 tbsps Soy Sauce Tamari
- 2 medium (approx 2-3/4" long, 2-1/2" dia) Sweet Red Peppers
- 2 cups chopped Broccoli
- 4 tbsps Natural Creamy Peanut Butter 1/3 Less Sodium & Sugar
- 1 1/2 fl ozs Lime Juice
- 3 tsps Chili Garlic Sauce
- 2 tsps Sucralose Based Sweetener (Sugar Substitute)
- 1/4 cup Cilantro (Coriander)

Directions
1. Preheat oven to 450°.
2. Combine 2 Tbsp tamari soy sauce and 2 Tbsp oil, set aside.

3. Cut tofu into 6 rectangles, brush with soy and oil mixture. Place on baking pan.
4. Add peppers and broccoli to baking pan and brush with soy and oil mixture. Bake for 10 minutes, turn tofu pieces over and continue to bake for an additional 12 minutes till tofu is browned and vegetables are softened.
5. While tofu and vegetable are baking, combine, peanut butter, lime juice, 1 Tbsp tamari, chili garlic sauce and sugar substitute in a sauce pan over low heat until warmed through.
6. Toss baked tofu and vegetables with sauce and serve immediately with cilantro on top.

Nutritional Information
- Protein : 38.5g
- Fat : 22.9g
- Fiber : 4.6g
- Calories :4.6g

Barbecue Rub

Servings: **12** | Prep: **5 m** | Style: **American**

Ingredients
- 2 tbsps Garlic Powder
- 2 tbsps Onion Powder
- 6 tsps Xylitol
- 1 1/2 tbsps Chili Powder
- 2 tbsps Cumin
- 1 1/2 tbsps Black Pepper
- 1 tsp Salt
- 1 tsp Yellow Mustard Seed

- 1 tsp Allspice Ground

Directions
1. Use this simple rub to spice up meats before grilling and roasting. Its flavor pairs beautifully with the Atkins recipe for Barbecue Sauce. Rub this on ribs before cooking and then baste the ribs with the sauce during the last 10-20 minutes of grilling or cooking. Each serving is 1 Tbsp.
2. Combine cumin, garlic powder, onion powder, xylitol, chili powder, pepper, salt, mustard and allspice in a bowl and mix well.
3. Rub onto ribs or other meats and marinate for at least an hour before grilling or baking. Remove rub before cooking and pat dry.
4. Rub lasts for up to a month in sealed container.

Nutritional Information
- Protein : 1.9g
- Fat : 16.2g
- Fiber : 2.9g
- Calories :22

Barbecue Sauce

Servings: 10 | **Prep:** 25 m | **Style**: American

Ingredients
- 1 tbsp Extra Virgin Olive Oil
- 1/4 cup chopped Onions
- 2 tbsps Tomato Paste
- 1 tsp Chili Powder
- 1 tsp Cumin

- 3/4 tsp Garlic Powder
- 3/4 tsp Yellow Mustard Seed
- 1/4 tsp Allspice Ground
- 1/8 tsp Red or Cayenne Pepper
- 1 1/2 cups Unsweetened Ketchup
- 1 tbsp Vinegar (Cider)
- 2/3 tbsp Worcestershire Sauce
- 2 tsps Sucralose Based Sweetener (Sugar Substitute)
- 1/4 tsp dry Coffee (Instant Powder)

Directions
1. Most commercial barbecue sauces are full of sugar or high-fructose corn syrup. Feel free to customize the sauce to your preferences or to the recipe you'll use this sauce with. For example, you can use more or less cayenne pepper or more or less vinegar as well as other spice combinations. Each serving is 2 scant Tbsp.
2. Heat oil in a medium saucepan over medium-high heat. Add onion and sauté until soft,
3. about 3 minutes.
4. Add tomato paste, chili powder, cumin, garlic powder, mustard, allspice and cayenne pepper, cook until fragrant, about 1 minute.
5. Stir in ketchup, vinegar, Worcestershire sauce, sugar substitute and coffee; simmer, stirring occasionally, until very thick, about 8 minutes.
6. Serve warm or at room temperature, or refrigerate in an airtight container for up to 3 days.

Nutritional Information
- Protein : 0.3g
- Fat : 1.5g
- Fiber : 0.3g

- Calories :32

Barbecued Glazed Ham

Servings: 10 | **Prep:** 25 m | **Style:** American | **Cook:** 90 m

Ingredients
- 80 oz boneless (yield after cooking) Fresh Ham
- 1 tbsp Chili Powder
- 1 tbsp Paprika
- 1 tsp Cumin
- 1/2 tsp Cinnamon
- 1/4 tsp Cloves (Ground)
- 1 tbsp Sucralose Based Sweetener (Sugar Substitute)
- 5 tbsps Sugar Free Apricot Preserves

Directions
1. Prepare the grill for indirect heat. Place a disposable aluminum drip pan in center of bottom grate or floor of grill. For a closed gas grill, heat on high for 10 to 15 minutes, then turn off heat source directly under pan, leaving the other one or two burners on. Adjust heat to register between 375°F and 425°F on an oven thermometer. For a charcoal grill, build two equal piles of briquettes on either side of drip pan. Burn coals about 25 minutes, until they are covered with gray ash.
2. Place ham onto grill and close lid. Grill 45 minutes. Turn ham over (adding more briquettes if necessary), and grill 45 to 60 minutes more, until an instant-read thermometer inserted in center of ham (away from bone) registers 140°F.
3. Combine chili powder, paprika, cumin, cinnamon, cloves and sugar substitute in a cup. Score top and sides of ham with a sharp knife in a crisscross pattern. Sprinkle rub over all sides.

4. Place ham on prepared grill over pan. Spoon or brush jam over ham. Cover and grill 5 minutes more. Let stand 15 minutes before carving.

Nutritional Information
- Protein : 43g
- Fat : 17.5g
- Fiber : 0.7g
- Calories :349

Basic Custard Ice Cream

Servings: 8 | **Prep:** 20 m | **Style:** American | **Cook:** 240 m

Ingredients
- 3 cups Heavy Cream
- 3 large Egg Yolks
- 1 large Egg (Whole)
- 3/4 cup Sucralose Based Sweetener (Sugar Substitute)
- 1/8 tsp Salt
- 1/2 tsp Vanilla Extract

Directions
1. In a medium heavy saucepan, heat cream until bubbles form just around the edge of the pan. Meanwhile, whisk together yolks, eggs, sugar substitute and salt.
2. Very slowly whisk the hot cream into the eggs. Pour the mixture back into the pan. Place over medium-low heat and cook, stirring constantly, just until the mixture thickens enough to coat the back of a spoon, 1 to 2 minutes.

3. Immediately remove from the heat and pour into a clean bowl. Stir in vanilla.
4. Cover the surface of the custard with plastic wrap and refrigerate until well chilled, about 4 hours. Freeze according to the directions for your ice cream maker.

Nutritional Information
- Protein : 3.6g
- Fat : 35.6g
- Fiber : 0g
- Calories :349

Basic Egg Salad

Servings: 4 | **Prep:** 5 m | **Style:** American

Ingredients
- 8 large Boiled Eggs
- 1/2 cup Real Mayonnaise
- 3 tsps Dijon Mustard
- 1/2 tsp Salt
- 1/4 tsp Black Pepper
- 2 stalk medium (7-1/2" - 8" long) Celery

Directions
1. Chop eggs roughly, or push them through the large-holed side of a four-sided box grater.
2. In a large mixing bowl, mix eggs with mayonnaise, mustard, salt and pepper with a wooden spoon. Stir in chopped celery.

3. Serve over lettuce or use low-carb bread or a tortilla to make a sandwich if you are in the correct phase and remember to add the extra grams to the total Net Carb count

Nutritional Information
- Protein : 12.6g
- Fat : 32.6g
- Fiber : 0.5g
- Calories :363

Basic Steamed Lobster With Drawn Butter

Servings: 4 | **Prep:** 5 m | **Style:** American | **Cook:** 15 m

Ingredients
- 4 lobsters Northern Lobster
- 3/4 cup Unsalted Butter Stick
- 1/2 fruit (2-1/8" dia) Lemon

Directions
1. Bring 10 quarts of salted water to a boil (you may need to use two pots).
2. Plunge lobsters directly into the boiling water, making sure they are completely covered. Bring the water back up to a boil. Cover and cook for 20 minutes from the time the water returns to a boil.
3. Remove lobsters from water with tongs; drain on paper towels.
4. Serve with butter in small dipping cups and lemon wedges.

Nutritional Information
- Protein : 28.6g
- Fat : 35.9g
- Fiber : 0.3g
- Calories :442

Basic Tomato Sauce

Servings: 6 | **Prep:** 10 m | **Style:** Italian | **Cook:** 30 m

Ingredients
- 1/4 cup Extra Virgin Olive Oil
- 1 medium (2-1/2" dia) Onions
- 1/2 stalk medium (7-1/2" - 8" long) Celery
- 2 cloves Garlic
- 1 tsp leaf Basil (Dried)
- 28 oz Crushed Tomatoes (Canned)

Directions
1. This versatile sauce is great not just with meatballs or on a low-carb or shirataki pasta, but also on sautéed zucchini, onions or peppers. Each serving is 1/2 cup.
2. Heat oil in a medium saucepan over medium heat. Dice the white onion, celery and garlic; add to pan and saute until the vegetables are very soft, about 6 minutes. Add basil and cook, stirring, 30 seconds.
3. Stir in tomatoes. Bring to a boil; reduce heat to medium-low and simmer, partially covered, until thickened, about 30 minutes. Season with salt and pepper. Serve hot

Nutritional Information
- Protein : 2.4g
- Fat : 9.7g
- Fiber : 2.8g
- Calories :128

Basil Pesto

Servings: 4 | **Prep:** 10 m | **Style:** Italian

Ingredients
- 6 oz Basil
- 1/3 cup Dried Pine Nuts
- 1/3 cup Parmesan Cheese (Grated)
- 1/2 tsp Garlic
- 1/2 tsp Salt
- 1/3 cup Extra Virgin Olive Oil

Directions
1. For this recipe you will need 3 cups of chopped basil. Despite its low carb content, this recipe is not appropriate for Induction because it contains nuts. Toasting the nuts enhances the flavor. Add more garlic if you prefer. Mix pesto with mayonnaise or cream cheese for a quick dip or thick sauce to spoon over fish, chicken, beef or steamed vegetables. It's also great atop slices of tomato and mozzarella. See variation below. Each servings is 1/4 cup.
2. Combine basil, pine nuts, Parmesan, garlic and salt in a food processor or blender; pulse until finely chopped.
3. Add oil in a slow and steady stream with machine running; process until fairly smooth but not puréed.

4. Serve immediately or refrigerate in an airtight container for up to 3 days or freeze for up to 1 month.
5. Arugula-Walnut Pesto: Prepare Basil Pesto according to directions, substituting arugula for the basil and walnuts for the pine nuts.

Nutritional Information
- Protein : 4.4g
- Fat : 24.6g
- Fiber : 5.4g
- Calories :258

Bearnaise Sauce

Servings: 8 | **Prep:** 10 m | **Style:** French | **Cook:** 10 m

Ingredients
- 2 tbsps chopped Shallots
- 1/2 tsp Tarragon
- 5 tbsps White Wine Vinegar
- 2 large Egg Yolks
- 1/2 cup Unsalted Butter Stick
- 1/8 tsp Salt
- 1/8 tsp Black Pepper

Directions
1. To make sauce: In a double boiler (or heatproof bowl set over, but not touching, a sauce pot of simmering water),

combine shallot, tarragon, and vinegar. Cook 5 minutes, until most of the vinegar has evaporated.
2. Whisk in egg yolk mixture. Whisk continuously until egg yolks have thickened, about 5 minutes. Whisk in butter gradually, piece by piece, until incorporated (sauce should have the texture of mayonnaise).
3. Remove from heat. Season to taste with salt and pepper.

Nutritional Information
- Protein : 0.9g
- Fat : 12.7g
- Fiber : 0g
- Calories :118

Béchamel Sauce

Servings: 6 | **Prep:** 10 m | **Style:** French | **Cook:** 20 m

Ingredients
- 1 cup Heavy Cream
- 1 cup Tap Water
- 2 tbsps chopped Onions
- 1 tsp Salt
- 1/8 tsp Black Pepper
- 1/8 tsp Nutmeg (Ground)
- 3 tsps Thick-It-Up
- 1 tbsp Unsalted Butter Stick

Directions

1. Béchamel is a mild sauce that can be used in soufflés or simmered with finely chopped vegetables or meats. Traditionally thickened with a mixture of flour and fat, our version uses heavy cream and a low-carb thickener instead. Each serving is 1/4 cup.
2. Combine cream, water, white onion, salt, pepper and nutmeg in a small saucepan over medium heat; bring to a simmer. Remove from heat; let stand for 15 minutes.
3. Strain cream mixture; return to saucepan over medium heat. Whisk in 1 tablespoon Thick-It-Up thickener; cook until sauce thickens, about 3 minutes.
4. Remove from heat; swirl in butter until melted. Use immediately

Nutritional Information
- Protein : 0.9g
- Fat : 16.7g
- Fiber : 1.1g
- Calories :163

Beef And Vegetable Stew

Servings: 6 | **Prep:** 10 m | **Style:** American | **Cook:** 165 m

Ingredients
- 1 1/2 lbs Beef Chuck (Mock Tender Steak, Lean Only, Trimmed to 1/4" Fat)
- 1 tsp leaf Dried Thyme Leaves
- 1 tsp leaf Oregano
- 1 tsp Rosemary (Dried)
- 1 tsp Paprika
- 2 tsps Salt
- 1 tsp Black Pepper

- 2 tbsps Extra Virgin Olive Oil
- 2 tbsps Unsalted Butter Stick
- 1 cup White Pearl Onions
- 2 cloves Garlic
- 16 fl ozs Merlot Wine
- 1 lb Green Snap Beans
- 1 medium Carrot
- 2 tbsps Thick-It-Up

Directions
1. Heat oven to 325°F.
2. Toss beef with thyme, oregano, rosemary, paprika, salt and pepper. Heat half the oil in a Dutch oven over medium-high heat. Brown half the beef; transfer to a bowl. Repeat with remaining oil and beef. Set aside.
3. Melt butter in Dutch oven or crock pot. Add onions; cook 7 8 minutes until onions begin to brown. Add garlic during last 2 minutes of cooking time.
4. Add reserved meat and accumulated juices, wine and 2 cups water. Bring to a boil. Cover Dutch oven and place in oven. Cook 2 hours, until beef is tender.
5. Add green beans and carrots; cook 15 minutes more, just until beans and carrots are tender.
6. Transfer Dutch oven to stove top over medium-high heat. Stir in thickener; cook 2 minutes more, stirring, until sauce thickens.
7. Adjust seasonings to taste and serve immediately.

Nutritional Information
- Protein : 23.3g
- Fat : 12.7g
- Fiber : 5g
- Calories :316

Beef Bolognaise With Parmesan

Servings: 6 | **Prep:** 10 m | **Style:** Italian | **Cook:** 25 m

Ingredients
- 1 1/2 lbs Beef Chuck (Mock Tender Steak, Lean Only, Trimmed to 1/4" Fat)
- 1 tsp leaf Dried Thyme Leaves
- 1 tsp leaf Oregano
- 1 tsp Rosemary (Dried)
- 1 tsp Paprika
- 2 tsps Salt
- 1 tsp Black Pepper
- 2 tbsps Extra Virgin Olive Oil
- 2 tbsps Unsalted Butter Stick
- 1 cup White Pearl Onions
- 2 cloves Garlic
- 16 fl ozs Merlot Wine
- 1 lb Green Snap Beans
- 1 medium Carrot
- 2 tbsps Thick-It-Up

Directions
1. Heat oven to 325°F.
2. Toss beef with thyme, oregano, rosemary, paprika, salt and pepper. Heat half the oil in a Dutch oven over medium-high heat. Brown half the beef; transfer to a bowl. Repeat with remaining oil and beef. Set aside.
3. Melt butter in Dutch oven or crock pot. Add onions; cook 7 8 minutes until onions begin to brown. Add garlic during last 2 minutes of cooking time.

4. Add reserved meat and accumulated juices, wine and 2 cups water. Bring to a boil. Cover Dutch oven and place in oven. Cook 2 hours, until beef is tender.
5. Add green beans and carrots; cook 15 minutes more, just until beans and carrots are tender.
6. Transfer Dutch oven to stove top over medium-high heat. Stir in thickener; cook 2 minutes more, stirring, until sauce thickens.
7. Adjust seasonings to taste and serve immediately.

Nutritional Information
- Protein : 27.1g
- Fat : 19.1g
- Fiber : 2.7g
- Calories :315

Beef Burger With Feta And Tomato

Servings: 4 | **Prep:** 10 m | **Style:** American| **Cook:** 12 m

Ingredients
- 1 lb Ground Beef (80% Lean / 20% Fat)
- 1 large Scallions or Spring Onion
- 1/2 cup Baby Spinach
- 1/4 cup chopped or sliced Red Tomatoes
- 1/4 cup crumbled Feta Cheese
- 1 1/2 tsps fresh Dill
- 1/2 tsp Salt
- 1/2 tsp Black Pepper

Directions

1. Combine ground beef, scallion, spinach, tomato, feta, 1.5 tsp fresh dill (or 1/2 tsp dried), salt and pepper. Form into 4 patties.
2. Grill or pan-fry over medium-high heat for 6 minutes per side for medium doneness.

Nutritional Information
- Protein : 24.3g
- Fat : 13.4g
- Fiber : 0.5g
- Calories :231

Beef Carpaccio With Arugula And Caper Vinaigrette

Servings: 6 | **Prep:** 15 m | **Style:** Italian

Ingredients
- 1 lb Ground Beef (80% Lean / 20% Fat)
- 1 large Scallions or Spring Onion
- 1/2 cup Baby Spinach
- 1/4 cup chopped or sliced Red Tomatoes
- 1/4 cup crumbled Feta Cheese
- 1 1/2 tsps fresh Dill
- 1/2 tsp Salt
- 1/2 tsp Black Pepper

Directions

1. Combine ground beef, scallion, spinach, tomato, feta, 1.5 tsp fresh dill (or 1/2 tsp dried), salt and pepper. Form into 4 patties.
2. Grill or pan-fry over medium-high heat for 6 minutes per side for medium doneness.

Nutritional Information
- Protein : 11.5g
- Fat : 19.7g
- Fiber : 0.3g
- Calories :226

Beef Fajitas With Peppers

Servings: 6 | **Prep:** 10 m | **Style:** Mexian | **Cook**: 10 m

Ingredients
- 1 1/2 tsps Garlic
- 1 tsp Salt
- 1 Jalapeno Pepper
- 2 tsps Cumin
- 3/4 cup Green Tomato Chile Sauce (Salsa Verde)
- 2 tbsps Extra Virgin Olive Oil
- 1 tbsp Canola Vegetable Oil
- 1 medium (approx 2-3/4" long, 2-1/2" dia) Red Sweet Pepper
- 1 small Red Onion
- 1 medium (approx 2-3/4" long, 2-1/2" dia) Green Sweet Pepper
- 1/4 cup Cilantro (Coriander)
- 12 tortillas Low Carb Tortillas

- 3/4 cup Sour Cream (Cultured)
- 1 fl oz Fresh Lime Juice
- 32 oz boneless (yield after cooking) Steak

Directions
1. Make marinade: In a large bowl or resealable plastic bag, combine garlic, salt, lime juice, jalapeno, cumin and olive oil; whisk together. Add steak pieces to marinade; coat well. Marinate, refrigerated at least 1 hour, preferably over night for the flavors to blend.
2. Heat oven to 350° F. Wrap tortillas in foil; place in oven to warm 15 minutes before serving.
3. Remove steak from marinade; discard marinade. Grill 5 inches over hot coals (or over medium-high heat) 3 to 4 minutes per side for medium-rare; set aside.
4. In a large skillet over medium-high heat, heat canola oil. Cook bell peppers and onion 5 minutes, until vegetables are softened.
5. Slice steak thinly across the grain.
6. To assemble fajitas, spread tortillas with salsa, top with steak slices and vegetable mixture, sour cream, and cilantro. Fold over and serve.

Nutritional Information
- Protein : 43.1g
- Fat : 30.5g
- Fiber : 10.3g
- Calories :507

Conclusion

The next step is, of course, to put the steps of the Atkins Diet into action! One cannot know what this type of diet can do for you if you only absorb its information without putting it to good use! From the contents of this book, you have learned the ways of the Atkins, how to incorporate it into your life without the hassle like other fad diets, and step by step, detailed instructions and delicious recipes that will get you quickly on your way to feeling much better about not only your appearance, but the way you feel on the inside as well.

Weight loss means making a change, and it is YOUR turn to take a turn for the better, to make the best of you even better than it currently is! Ensure that you are making this encouraged change for yourself, because even if you lose your goal weight, it is still what's on the inside that matters the most! But, let's be honest, looking good on the outside will certainly keep those bad thoughts that you have about yourself on a daily basis at bay! Good luck in your weight loss quest!

www.ingramcontent.com/pod-product-compliance
Lightning Source LLC
Chambersburg PA
CBHW071439070526
44578CB00001B/142